I0437712

The Weight Loss HandBook

The Weight Loss Handbook

Your Quick Guide to Total Success!

By

WEIGHT LOSS AND LIFE TRANSFORMATION
COACH: **EFTHYMIOS TZIMAS**

iUniverse, Inc.
Bloomington

The Weight Loss Handbook
Your Quick Guide to Total Success!

Copyright © 2011 by Efthymios Tzimas.

All rights reserved. No part of this book may be used or reproduced by any means, graphic, electronic, or mechanical, including photocopying, recording, taping or by any information storage retrieval system without the written permission of the publisher except in the case of brief quotations embodied in critical articles and reviews.

You should not undertake any diet/exercise regimen recommended in this book before consulting your personal physician. Neither the author nor the publisher shall be responsible or liable for any loss or damage allegedly arising as a consequence of your use or application of any information or suggestions contained in this book.

iUniverse books may be ordered through booksellers or by contacting:

iUniverse
1663 Liberty Drive
Bloomington, IN 47403
www.iuniverse.com
1-800-Authors (1-800-288-4677)

Because of the dynamic nature of the Internet, any web addresses or links contained in this book may have changed since publication and may no longer be valid. The views expressed in this work are solely those of the author and do not necessarily reflect the views of the publisher, and the publisher hereby disclaims any responsibility for them.

Any people depicted in stock imagery provided by Thinkstock are models, and such images are being used for illustrative purposes only.
Certain stock imagery © Thinkstock.

ISBN: 978-1-4620-2451-3 (sc)
ISBN: 978-1-4620-2452-0 (hc)
ISBN: 978-1-4620-2453-7 (ebk)

Library of Congress Control Number: 2011916847

Printed in the United States of America

iUniverse rev. date: 11/03/2011

Contents

A message from your coach:

Life in its self is a gift from God. To live life to your fullest potential and happiness is your thank you!

Best of Luck! You may send me a message or check out my webpage at efthymiostzimas@gmail.com

Dedication

This book is dedicated to:

I would like to dedicate this book to my wife Efi. Thank you for all your love and emotional support. You are a daily breath of fresh air and the fullness of my heart. If our love is forever, than eternal, are we!

Preface

Welcome to the world of total success. Today is a special day. Your decision to take action and control the quality of your life is one of courage and dedication. How many times have we all heard the words I should have or I could have etc. coming from the mouth of our loved ones and friends? In many cases its heart breaking and there really are no words to help ease the suffering and emptiness that one feels when they reach a part of their lives where circumstances limit their passion for life. The time to act is now. You will learn key principals needed to kick start areas of your life that are limiting your total success. You will learn fundamentals about how habits are formed and how to change habits that will lead you down a path of growth instead of limitation.

The day will come when you will be a driving force for your family and loved ones. You must believe in yourself and decide to take action on a daily basis to achieve a transformation that will become a solid foundation of character over a short period of time. You will become healthier, stronger, smarter and better overall as your accomplishments; stack up one upon another thru out your life. Believe in yourself and have faith as you now are not alone but have me next to you as your coach. You will be totally successful if you chose to be. This is your beginning. Let's begin together, starting now!

Biography

Permit me to introduce myself. My name is Efthymios Tzimas. I was born in Greece. My parents brought me to America when I was just months in age and a new born. Since the beginning I had excess weight and struggled in life from early childhood with my appearance and my weight. Children can be cruel with name calling and other forms of abuse especially in a country that basis such focus on appearances. Well, as you can imagine that my character and habits were created within myself under the principals of fight or flight. I remember how food became such an addiction and how it eased my pain and suffering as I suffered the cruel abuses in life because of my body and appearance. I started getting bigger by the month and the child grew up to become a young adult weighing in at his peak a whopping 462 pounds.

This was 22 years ago and I have lost over 268 pounds. I have lost and kept off all the weight and have been fluctuating from 180 to 190 pounds ever since. Now for 20 years I have been training and motivating people just like you to change the areas of their lives starting with their health and appearance. I am internationally certified as a nutritional coach and fitness expert. I challenge you now to seize the day and believe in yourself first and then in me as your coach that all things in life are possible as long as you believe, have faith and act. Let's agree now that there is no tomorrow and no past but the actions of today and every day from now on that determine your destiny. Your future and the new you awaits you.

Your Story

Please feel free to write to us and tell us about your results. Share your story and success with us with e-mail and visit us on our web page at: efthymiostzimas@gmail.com

Warning: Please check with and get cleared by a licensed physician before starting and participating in any exercise program, nutritional food plan and or diet:

INDIVIDUAL RESULTS WILL VARY!

Introduction

Congratulations. My name is Efthymios Tzimas and I am your personal weight loss coach and fitness trainer. I lost 268 pounds and have kept the excess weight off for over twenty years. In this work book, or should I say, your guide to all accomplishments, you will find your breath of fresh air and your sword to all success. With obesity, which is spreading worldwide like a plague, it is easy at times to fall into the traps of giving up, becoming discouraged and failing to accomplish your weight loss goal. You must not utilize crash diets or a strictly low caloric diet as your weapon to succeed. Crash diets and very low caloric diets do not work. These diets provide the body with temporary results and are accomplished through the use of human will power, which we all now know, provides you with temporary results or a quick fix. Everything in life that is permanent requires a formula if you will, for success. Here it is. First we need to make a conscious decision and have clarity about what we are seeking to gain. Then we need to get our game plan together. The game plan is actions taken on a daily basis that drive you closer to your goal. After a period of time you then receive the fruits of your labor known as change. Decisions plus Actions equal Change. This is the formula to all success in life. Not only for over coming obesity permanently, but for all transformation and accomplishments that are desired in your present and future.

With the disease of obesity it is easy to fall into the traps of discouragement and failure. To let crash diets burn you out time and time again. To let a scale manipulate your strength and mood according to what number it shows you daily. Imagine, you weigh your success or failures according to a reading that is false most of the times and this reading, manipulates your mood. This scale, tells you if you are a failure or if you have success. A lifeless machine that is wrong most of the times has a power to control your emotional state and feelings. Let's decide right now to throw our scales in the garbage where they belong. To go through life and be guided by the way we feel, our internal health and wellbeing and the way we look concerning fat to muscle ratios. You may even use your clothes as a guide or buy smaller clothes or the sizes you want to fit in and use them as motivation and your final reward will be you fitting into them. However a scale is garbage and it belongs there, in the garbage. I want to briefly remind out that the mind is the most powerful weapon we possess and we need to use it in a positive and productive manner. There is no room for self-doubt or fear. There is no room for past failures however we can recall our past successes. It is in both that our lessons in life are learned and our characteristics beliefs are developed. We've all heard the phrases it's all in the mind or if knowledge was power than a God am I.

Well I regret to inform you that knowledge is only powerful when used in a positive manner for yourself and all humanity. What good is knowledge without action? The result is the same. Failure! Knowledge works hand in hand with action once a decision is made. Then and only then, can a permanent transformation or change occur.

As a child I always found myself to be heavier than all the other children my age. What guided me was an appetite that was not easily satisfied. I was able to eat uncontrollably and I was always hungry. I can't remember how many times I vomited as a child because my body couldn't hold the amounts of food I was giving it. Family members saw no fault in this hunger. It was believed that I needed all this food so that I may grow up in height and in stature. I became strong and powerful. Well as you can imagine, I did grow up to be tall and strong with a fifty four inch waist. I was very powerful yet I suffered every day as I was growing up. My problem was not just that I couldn't find clothes as I was growing up, but I suffered in the hands of all others criticism including my family members. I was made fun of all the time and talked about. I was the joke for most and received full attention as there criticism flowed out of their mouths and hearts. I received the wrong type of attention of course. The kids and even adults tend to be harsh and quick with their tongues and criticisms.

There words, laughter and the way they looked at me and judged me, helped me sink into the depths of my own spirit where I hid and ate and became unsociable. Life became very lonely and eating food while watching TV was indeed, my best friend. That had become the ultimate fix for me. Eating and watching TV. What a destructive combo yet a quick escape from my reality into a world or a life that was not mine. Food always made me feel better when I was eating it however I felt anger and betrayal, weakness and disgust in myself after I was done eating and my trip in TV land was done. Suddenly reality sneaks in and I have gained more weight and have lost from my self-respect and dignity for myself, once again. This vicious cycle continued until one day I said enough. I will either live my life the way I want under my control or I am going to die trying. I will not die like this and be buried in a piano case. I refuse to not have control over myself in every area of my life. I made a decision and then I acted out my plan as I accomplished change daily.

You now know how food becomes an addictive drug as it provides a temporary fix of pleasure. These wrong actions over a period of time since childhood were the destructive force driving me to an early grave as the calories contributed to my obesity. By taking the wrong repeated actions over a period of time I programmed myself. I linked the wrong associations in my mind and linked pain and pleasure to the wrong principals and stimuli. Our actions shape and define our character, our appearance and our health both mentally and physically.

In your guide/work book you will receive the tools, the understanding and a simpler way of looking at things and reprograming old habits with new ones. You will have a better understanding of why you feel the way you do and why you do the things you do. You will change your lives and break your old habits by reprograming into your subconscious mind new responses to the same stimuli over period of time. Then your new actions will wipe out old habits as new habits are now formed. Whether it is a psychological factor or just a need to consume fewer calories, you now have the tools necessary to become happier, healthier and more positive in all areas of your life. Now the time has come for you to understand the true factors that have caused you to retreat into the depths of yourself, while feeling trapped and in bondage. Almost as if you are living a life that is not yours and is a participant in a very bad dream. It is a survival mechanism to retreat into once self when pain is offered to you daily. However this retreat leads down a path of even worse problems and a very low self-esteem. The time has come to decide and act. Grab your sword and fight. Let's go. Tomorrow is not promised to anyone. Live for the day but live as you truly want. The time for change is now and I am with you.

Let's go fight, our lives are worth it!

MY CONSIDERATIONS FOR A HEALTHIER WEIGHT ACCORDING TO BONE FRAMES FOR MEN AND WOMEN.

AVERAGES FOR A WOMAN

Height without shoes and suggested pounds for small, medium and large bone frames.

5 feet 0 inches	—	96-131 pounds
5 feet 1 inches	—	98-132 pounds
5 feet 2 inches	—	104-134 pounds
5 feet 3 inches	—	107-139 pounds
5 feet 4 inches	—	115-145 pounds
5 feet 5 inches	—	118-150 pounds
5 feet 6 inches	—	122-152 pounds
5 feet 7 inches	—	129-155 pounds
5 feet 8 inches	—	130-156 pounds
5 feet 9 inches	—	133-158 pounds
5 feet 10 inches	—	140-160 pounds
5 feet 11 inches	—	142-162 pounds
6 feet 0 inches	—	145-165 pounds

AVERAGES FOR A MAN

Height without shoes and suggested pounds for a small, medium and large bone frames.

5 feet 4 inches	—	126-158 pounds
5 feet 5 inches	—	127-160 pounds
5 feet 6 inches	—	132-163 pounds
5 feet 7 inches	—	134-165 pounds
5 feet 8 inches	—	139-166 pounds
5 feet 9 inches	—	141-168 pounds
5 feet 10 inches	—	145-174 pounds
5 feet 11 inches	—	150-176 pounds
6 feet 0 inches	—	162-185 pounds
6 feet 1 inches	—	165-190 pounds
6 feet 2 inches	—	168-195 pounds
6 feet 3 inches	—	170-200 pounds
6 feet 4 inches	—	174-204 pounds
6 feet 5 inches	—	178-210 pounds
6 feet 6 inches	—	180-215 pounds
6 feet 7 inches	—	185-220 pounds

BELIEVE IN YOURSELF AS I BELIEVE IN YOU

Welcome. Let's start off with our game plan. We made the decision to lose weight and change the quality of our life. You have hired a leading expert and coach in the area of health and fitness by buying this hand book, as your first action. What's your next step? The game plan, or your plan of execution based on your decision to change a specific area of your life in great clarity. Let's get a clear picture with conscious thought, about what it is that we want to accomplish both physically and mentally in the area of our life that we are now focused on to change. Grab a pen or pencil and let's put in writing our plan of execution. Clarity is very important. The reasons you want to change and the end results will be your reality until you accomplish your goal. What we focus on daily and our conscious thoughts, is our reality and our life as a whole. Clarity is very important and a direct plan that involves detail. Let's start now by making our schedule and our plan on how we will accomplish our goals on a daily basis. What actions should we take and what thoughts shall we entertain?

Let's begin our day every morning with the following thoughts. Today is my day to fight and conquer. Tomorrow is not promised to anyone what counts is what I do today. Inspire yourself daily. Hear the warrior that we all have deep inside. Hear your voice and release your strength.

When you listen to the warrior inside you face life with power and you flee from nothing yet conquer all things you focus on. Be a leader of your on life and live by example. Others will see your actions and you will be known to all observers. The warrior voice inside that we all have, cries out for justice and power. You may have heard others call it positive thinking. Maybe you have heard others say: think positive and not negative. This is the voice of fight and not flight. Sooner or later we must face our enemy and fight because if we keep fleeing we will sooner or later become a victim of our on circumstance. Avoid negative situations and negative people. These words and sayings have been handed down throughout the generations for a reason. Negativity leads to misery, loss, bitterness and death. Positivity leads to life and fullness. The people that usually affect one's life in a negative way are all the people we allow. This includes ourselves with wrong habits and our friends, family members and loved ones. They are the closest to us and 99 percent of the time our defenses are down when they are around us. There words and looks seep into us like a sponge because of our comfort zone and our lack of defense when we are around them. Put up your defenses and be aware of what you are mentally observing. Have a voice and agree to disagree. Be a leader and develop your own character of respect. Followers live a difficult life and a leader lives a life of gain and respect. Think about this very carefully.

How many times did you listen to the wrong person and took the wrong actions instead of hearing your own voice? If I were to guess I would say that 95 percent of the time you were right and you should have listened to yourself and they were wrong. If you don't know what's best for you, than who does? All advice given by others has to do with their lives and the things they have seen and experienced. Don't forget the magic word here is they have seen in their lives. Do you understand? Their life is not yours. Be a leader there are enough followers in the world. Listen to yourself and the warrior inside that cries out for justice, mercy and leadership. I have every faith in you and I know you can accomplish anything you set your mind to. Take action! Write down on a piece of paper or your work book your decisions and the actions that are necessary to live the life you so desperately desire. Today is a new day. Today all things of the past are forgotten and all things have become new. You are a new person with new actions. Let's start the day with a sample menu. Start with breakfast and while you are eating strategize the day's actions and your goals for the day including your exercise routine that should be no less than 40 minutes. Write down your road map for the day so that you may execute the actions that are necessary to accomplish for that day. Remember that it will be the daily executions of these actions that will accomplish your changes.

These actions will lead you closer every day to your success and your new reality as the new person is formed and shaped by your own hand. There is no tomorrow just the actions and your daily plan as you create it daily at breakfast. Don't be distracted and follow the plan. Your road map for success is before you. Have faith and believe in yourself. Never let others tell you otherwise. Live your life with 100 percent commitment to yourself and your daily plan. By doing so, after a period of time you would have become a leader and others will live by your example and accomplishments. Remember, negative people will always be around you. Always be careful on what you agree with and what you accept from others. Others ideas thoughts negative emotions and weaknesses can become a poison if you choose to consume it. You don't want to wake up one morning when your older and greyer and say to yourself, I should have done this or I could have done that. Seize the day. Every day that goes by does not come back. Don't waste it. Life is to precious so decide right now that you will never waste it in misery and bondage again. Break these chains of bondage that you yourself have created through time by take the wrong actions. You have programmed yourself by taking actions consistently to be at a point of your life that is unpleasing. Every day is precious and it's a fresh new opportunity and a start. If you don't succeed one day, don't give up just start again. I believe your worth the fight. Never give up on your decisions and never give up on yourself.

I never will give up on you as I believe in you. Not because I know you but because I was you. If I can change my life, everyone can. Throughout my 20 years of coaching and training my worst student was myself. That's why I say that if I can do it everyone can. Never give up on yourself, your life is too precious. Live it with no limitations and a desire to be the real you. If you don't act on your own, I have learned that no one will do it for you. Have faith and believe in your daily actions. You may not be able to see your results daily, but believe you me they are happening and over a period of time you will be amazed and happy with your end results. Others who do not see you daily will notice changes and a transformation. Have faith and believe. Take action and bring your decisions to life. After a period of time you will have accomplished extraordinary changes. Then you will finally breathe and live as the real you, the person you have always dreamed of. No excuses and no bondages. I know you can do it! This is your new beginning. I am honored to be your coach!

UNDERSTANDING FOODS.

Foods are broken down into 3 major categories.

Carbohydrates:

1. **Complex carbohydrates.**
   Examples:
   A) Rice, Pasta, Potatoes etc.

2. **Simple Carbohydrates.**
   Examples:
   B) Fruits, Sugar & Vegetables.

Proteins:

Examples:
A) Red Meat, Poultry, Egg Whites and Fish.

Fats:

Examples:
Animal fats, Oils, Butter and Cheeses etc.

Things To Avoid:

Animal Fat, Oils, Butters and Margarines, Junk Foods, Fast Foods, Cheeses, Whole Milk, Sugars and Salts.

CARBOHYDRATES: Energy at its best!

Simple Carbohydrates.

1. Simple carbohydrates are as the word states. Simple. The body has the ability to simply break down the simple carbohydrates, (food) into fuel faster than any other type of food source. Take for example sugar. This simple carbohydrate can instantly be used by the body with such speed that sugar can be administered under the tongue in its natural form, and will be absorbed into the blood stream. How is that for simple and fast?

2. Simple carbohydrates consist of 4 calories per gram of consumption.

3. Simple carbohydrates are broken down faster and provide the body with a faster source of energy. The main function of the stomach is to break down all food and prep it for absorption as it passes thru the intestinal track.

4. Good examples of these simple carbohydrates are fruit and vegetables. Even though sugars are an immediate source of energy, they are not a stable source. Sugars will give you a peak or immediate boost of energy and then drop your energy peak as you crash to a low or instant feeling of being tired. These peaks and crashes are not good for your heart and can affect your glucose levels, the body's stabilization of energy and even blood pressure, in a negative way.

5. Choose vegetables and fruit. Up to 3 fruits a day is a very wise choice over all. Especially if choosing grapefruits and apples as your fruit choices. Vegetables can be eaten unlimitedly. You may cook them or steam them and even eat most of them raw. Simple carbohydrates provide you with vitamins, minerals, some fiber and a stable, constant stream of energy. Try to avoid adding toppings to them so that you make keep your calories lower. Eat them as simple and as natural as you possibly can.

Phrases To Remember:

I eat to live and NOT live to eat!
A calorie avoided is a calorie burned and earned.
If you eat it, you must burn it.
If you don't use it you will wear it.
Never eat when you're tired.

CARBOHYDRATES: ENERGY AT ITS BEST!

Carbohydrates are broken down into 2 categories. Complex Carbohydrates and Simple Carbohydrates.

Complex Carbohydrates:

1. Complex Carbohydrates are a fuel source that are broken down and released into the blood stream as they are needed by the body. They provide a stable form of energy that can be used for a longer period of time. The body needs more time to break them down and make them available for energy.
2. Complex Carbohydrates have a nutritional value of 4 calories per gram.
3. Examples of Complex Carbohydrates are: Pasta, rice, potatoes, etc.
4. The body breaks down Complex Carbohydrates into a longer lasting more stable form of energy. This is the best form of energy for every athlete no matter what the sport of choice is.

PROTEIN AT ITS BEST!

Protein is a requirement not a choice. Protein is used for muscular strength and repair. Protein provides the body with the necessary building blocks and amino acids, that will help your body mend, build and develop your working muscles. Without the adequate amounts of protein, an athlete will find it extremely difficult to add muscle and repair working muscles as recuperation will take much longer. Without protein you shouldn't lift weights and over exert yourself because your work out will be wasted. especially if you are lifting weights. Training with weights requires an adequate amount of protein and rest to fully benefit from your workout. Any physical exertion and muscular injuries, tears or breakdown of muscle tissue that occurs during the day, requires protein to build and heal those muscles. Without protein, any exertion and injuries would take a very long time to heal and you would be in constant pain over a longer period of time depending on the stress and damage caused to your muscle structure. No protein means, no gain in muscle, no strength and no repaired recuperation. A good rule of thumb for every athlete is a gram of protein per pound of body weight especially when weights and physical sports are involved. There is a saying that states, if you don't use your muscles you will lose them.

Without protein even if you use the muscles you will still lose them and not benefit from your exercise to the fullest. Remember that overall health and fitness is your main goal.

The best form of protein will come from egg whites. Egg whites are very low in calories with no fat. The best sources of protein are as follows in the order I have listed them. Egg whites, chicken breast, broiled meat and last but not least is fish. All other foods might have traces of protein and some vegetables do have more protein than others however they do not supply the body with the building blocks necessary to achieve maximum muscular development. That is why in cases of a vegetarian, an athlete must include branched chain amino acids in there nutritional program. Please remember that protein and a great source of it is a requirement for every athlete and everybody. Muscles need protein for repairs and to develop. To keep the calories low and as fat free as possible, you can broil the protein, boil it or grill it. Avoid frying the protein as much as possible. By not doing so your protein will provide your body with more pluses and very few minuses. Think of protein as muscle and muscle as protein. An athlete can't have one without the other. Get stronger, faster and leaner by not forgetting adequate amounts of protein and rest to go along with your workouts.

Take advantage of this 3 part combination and your results will be outstanding. Protein, rest and exercise is the secret for every athlete and every person for muscular development and recuperation. Add carbohydrates to the formula and you now have the fuel. This is the secret to all physical development and body transformations. Remember; keep all your meals as low fat as possible. Drink eight to ten glasses of water a day. Exercise and consume adequate amounts of protein for muscular development and recuperation. Eat carbohydrates so that you may have fuel for the muscles to work and get plenty of rest. Keep your meals as low fat as possible and you now control your caloric counts and burn fat. You will do great! Let's now move on to the next part of your work book that will be giving you a better understanding of food.

UNDERSTANDING FOODS:

FATS: SOME ARE GOOD MOST ARE BAD!

Fats.

1. All foods today have a caloric count usually listed on the outside wrapping included in everything we buy to eat and drink. This is a great help when we are counting calories. Fat has a higher caloric count than protein and carbohydrates. For 1 gram of protein and carbohydrate you consume 4 calories. For 1 gram of fat you consume 9 calories. Mathematically that is more than twice the amounts of calories than a gram of protein or a gram of carbohydrates. That is a significant amount of calories if you love fatty foods and fried foods. If you keep your fat consumption low you can actually eat more food and still lose weight or at least maintain your weight. Think about this in terms of arithmetic. More fat means more calories and less health.

2. Fats for example are nutrients that are not good for you, especially animal fat. Fat holds cholesterol and a higher caloric count. Even though some fats are necessary for healthy skin and hair, for example nuts, you should avoid animal fats and cheeses as much as possible.

3. Fats are found mostly in products that contain proteins which are derived from animals. Examples: Meats, chicken, fish, whole milk, cheeses and yogurts. This fat content found in animals is stored energy as it is in humans. They are nothing but extra calories stored around weak muscles. It is around weak and unused muscles where fat is stored in human beings as well as in animals. You will find fat cells layered under the skin with water and it covers the muscles. Even though this extra fat can keep you warmer especially people living in cold temperatures, it hinders the proper body functions and circulation. Excess fat puts pressure on the skeleton, joints and the spinal column. It thickens the blood causing blood pressure to rise because the heart needs to work harder to circulate food and nutrients and the cholesterol in the blood layers the inside and outside of your organs as well as thickening your arteries. This causes you a lack of energy and many health problems over all. It has been proven that fat is the major cause of strokes and heart failure, once the artery walls

are blocked and layered with cholesterol worldwide. Imagine how dangerous it is since heart failure is the number one killer worldwide. Let's avoid animal fat as much as possible.

4. Fat has a nutritional value of 9 calories per gram consumed. In other words, if you eat more fat you need to work harder per gram consumed to burn it off. The higher the fat you consume the greater the chances your body storing it and not burning it off.

5. Fat is the last form of energy the body will use. Most of the time the body will just store it as extra calories. As we now know that stored calories in every form is another name for fat. However animal fats all provide cholesterol and other bad nutrients that are not necessary for the body and affect overall health.

6. There are foods that have natural fat. Some of these fats are needed for healthy hair, nails and skin. However even these foods need to be eaten in moderation. They benefit the body and provide some of our needed fiber. These fats are found in nuts for example and yogurts. Yogurts do have other benefits like enzymes that help the body with digestion and to fight off bacteria. These foods should be eaten with moderation but animal fats and cheeses and whole milk are not needed nor are they necessary for overall health. If you need to you can add a multi vitamin instead.

7. For a healthier and slimmer new you, think low fat. It's definitely the best way to go over all.

8. Please remember that fat is a poor choice of energy and the body would much rather store it than break it down to use as energy. There are much better choices that the body would prefer to use as energy and that are carbohydrates.

9. Keep your fat content low and your energy levels high. A low fat diet is the cause of a longer, healthier and more productive life. A low fat diet allows your energy levels to be higher and more stable and your organs work smoother and better without added stress.

UNDERSTANDING THE MAJOR FUNCTIONS OF PROTEINS, CARBOHYDRATES AND FATS.

Carbohydrates:

1. Complex carbohydrates have a time released affect in the body. They are released and used as needed throughout the day.
2. Simple carbohydrates provide a much quicker supply of energy to be used.

* Simple Carbohydrates are digested much faster by the body.

Protein:

1. Protein is used by the body to repair muscles and organ tissue as they are worked daily.
2. Protein is also used by the muscles to get stronger and bigger as athletes purposely break there muscle tissue down and utilize protein and branched chain amino acids for muscular growth during adequate rest states.

*Basically think of protein as muscle and muscle as protein.

Fat:

1. Fat is also energy but not a good source.
2. Fat is the last form of energy the body will use. Most of the time the body will just store it as extra calories. As we know stored calories are another name for fat.

* All foods have natural fat. This fat is needed for many of the bodily functions. It is the extra fat and cholesterol that the body does not need that is usually consumed when eating meats, cheeses and milk products.

Healthy Tip:

When cooking food and while eating, use natural fat burners that burn fat and lower cholesterol. These natural fat burners are lemons, vinegar, onions and garlic. Try to cook your food with these natural fat burners and eat them daily. Another natural fat burner is the grapefruit. You can actually lose anywhere from 5 pounds and greater just by eating one a day over the course of one year.

DUMPING THE GARBAGE:

Important: You must decide that certain foods are to be limited in your life from now on to ensure overall health and fitness.
These foods are:

1. Sugar
2. Salt
3. Oil
4. Animal Fat
5. Butter
6. Margarine
7. All Junk Foods
8. Flower
9. Regular Sodas
10. Whole Milk
11. Excess nuts
12. Cheeses
13. Fried Foods and Fast Food
14. Cakes including chocolate and creams
15. Hard Liquor and beers

DUMPING THE GARBAGE
CONTINUED:

Use this list as substitutions for the foods to be avoided as much as possible.

1. Sugar Substitute
2. Pepper
3. Pam Light Cooking Sprays
4. Light Popcorn
5. Light Beer
6. Diet Soda
7. Fat Free or low fat Milk or Soy
8. Fat Free or low fat Cheese or Soy
9. Broiled Foods
10. Veggie Products
11. Soy Products
12. Olive Oil
13. Apple Sauce with no added sugar. Example: For Baking
14. Dark Chocolate
15. All Natural Fruit and Vegetable Drinks.

EXAMPLES OF PLATE COMBINATIONS:

1. For the first month your plate should have the following ratios and your food consumed accordingly.

2. 50% Carbohydrates, 30% Proteins, 20% Fats.

3. For the second month your plate should have the following ratios and your food consumed accordingly.

4. 55% Carbohydrates, 30% Proteins, 15% Fats.

5. For the third month and every month after, your plate should have the following ratios and your food consumed accordingly.

6. 60% Carbohydrates, 30% Proteins, 10% Fats.

*Remember: Carbohydrates are our fuel source. They provide us with energy. The better quality the fuel source, the healthier and stronger our body is and works throughout the day. Fat clogs the arteries and decreases the flow of fuel to the heart, organs and muscle tissue. All muscles and organs skin and blood need protein for repairs and for the development of strength and endurance. Combine proteins, carbohydrates together with limitations of fat, get sleep, exercise, water, soluble fiber and a multi vitamin and you will gain health.

PHYSICAL ACTIVITIES FOR MIND, BODY TRANSFORMATION AND STRESS RELIEF:

Examples:

1. Go to the movies. If you can walk to your destination it is even better.
2. Go shopping. Buy clothes you love, that are smaller in size so that you may target fitting into them in the near future. This tactic will motivate you and push you harder to succeed.
3. Go out with friends and family members that are positive and inspiring.
4. Go for long walks to clear your mind.
5. Join in physical games and sports that are being played. Baseball, soccer, volleyball, handball, football, water polo e
6. Go jogging or a run or choose power walking.
7. Write your thoughts and feelings along with long and short term goals on paper or use recording devices to capture moments of thoughts and plans. This will help you notice changes in your emotions and thoughts as occurrences unfold daily in your life. This way you can go into your journal or recording device and remember or revisit your thoughts and responses as you faced occurrences and changes throughout different moments and days in your life. You then will be able to make changes to your initial responses as new stimuli or similar stimuli occur.
8. Take up martial art classes.
9. Take up classes that require thought and physical actions. These classes require creativity and imagination for example: Painting, pottery, art, creative writing, acting, singing etc.
10. Take classes that can teach to do work around the house or build and repair thing.

Hint: Occupy your mind and body with new and inspiring things that will help shape and refine the new you. Change is a great and exciting thing which breathes new life into a person and an old routine. It helps build new habits and character which will be a foundation for the new you.

THE ROLE OF EXERCISE

IMPORTANT: (Check with your doctor before starting any weight loss system, diet and or exercise program. It is highly recommended that you get cleared by your doctor after a full blood test and cardiac/ stress test is done.)

Exercise is very important for a healthy body and a clear mind. When the muscles of the body are used or stressed, they force the body to work at a different and higher level of energy expenditure utilizing more calories as the calories are transformed into fuel for the working muscles. The body is made to be used but not abused to handle different levels of physical stress and to deliver different energy outputs as long as it is trained to do so over a period of time. The problem that most of us face is that we get stuck or used to a daily routine that usually involves no exercise. These daily routines keep the body used to a regular energy output and does not stimulate a faster metabolism but instead, it slows down our metabolic rate. Metabolism is the body's ability to utilize or burn the calories given on a daily basis. Some people can burn food faster than others on a normal basis without exercise and others can't. There are 2 forms of metabolism. The first form is called anabolism. Anabolism is when the body is in the state of weight gain and a desire or hunger for more food.

The other state is called catabolism. Catabolism is the state of the body which it loses weight. Our goal is to force the body to change from the anabolism state which is weight gain to a catabolic state which is weight loss. After that we want to be able to maintain our weight. To make it simple just think that the calories consumed daily will keep you at a specific weight. Let's suppose that you want to maintain a weight of 160 pounds, than your daily goal is 1600 calories a day. Basically take your desired weight and add a zero to it. That would be your daily caloric count and target. Exercise is the shock principal needed to break the body out of an anabolic state and force it along with a lower calorie menu, into a catabolic state known as weight loss. Once the weight is lost than you maintain your caloric intake for the day. Exercise is the shock principal that stimulates and forces the body into a higher level of energy expenditure which provides you over a period of time with more endurance. This shock principal causes the body to burn more calories faster, so that the muscles may keep up with the minds command for contraction and movement. At first all new stimulants are rejected by the body and mind because change is usually not welcomed and the body and mind will try to reject anything new including a change in food and exercise. Remember that no one welcomes change once they are stuck in habits and a routine that is comfortable to them.

However as all habits are formed and routines over a period of time, utilizing repetition, so will new habits be formed over a length of time. It will be just a matter of repetition and taking new action. Even though it will be uncomfortable at first the body will learn new things and get into new routines as new habits are formed to deliver the success you so desperately deserve.

Exercise is needed by the body to start losing weight or burn fat and for development of muscle tissue and endurance. You need to start using up more calories on a weekly basis than you are consuming in order to stop anabolism and force the body into a catabolic state. Exercise forces the body to tap into your fat cells for the extra calories you are not giving it. The fat cells than release the stored fat or extra calorie so that the body can keep up with the demand of fuel. As the fat cells deliver or release this stored energy, they become smaller. As they shrink your bodies form changes and because these fat cells have less stored energy so they shrink. That is how you lose inches and weight. As these fat cells shrink they release extra water as well. Under the skin we have fat cells that are blown up and a layer of water pressed together under the skin. The fat cell shrinks and the extra water is then released. The water retention or bloat goes away and the fat cells shrink. When this occurs you have just gone down a size or lost weight. Exercise is needed by the body to lose weight and water retention and to burn fat. It makes your process of change occur faster as you become healthier on the inside.

Please do not burn yourself out by over exercising and by starving yourself. This will do more harm than good and in the process you will lose more muscle than fat. Starvation diets do not work and if change occurs it will be temporary and not permanent. When you starve yourself the body is forced into a survival mode. It starts using more of your own muscle as food and reserves the fat for the future because it feels that you might not give it the food necessary for survival. The body falls into a survival mode and starts shutting down as if you were to hibernate or sleep for a season. Then energy levels drop tremendously, which can cause headaches, dizziness, mood swings but most of all anger as your body goes under tremendous shocks during your starvation or survival mode. It is in our genes to survive and a subconscious response to self-preserve. That is why we must avoid starvation diets and by doing so we avoid having low energy and drops in our blood sugar levels that cause dizziness. Let's not forget the unnecessary stress put on our hearts and organs to stay alive. Starvation diets or crash diets are to be avoided no matter how great the temptation. Exercise and counting calories is the best way to go. No short cuts and no magic pills or medicine. None of these things are permanent. Even surgeries the cut out portions of the stomach or have a ring placed around the stomach, provide for temporary results.

The reason is first we have not changed our way of thinking by forming new habits thru new repeated actions and because the stomach is an expandable bag which can grow again and expand further. There are no short cuts in life and nothing worth having comes overnight or without work and effort. Start by exercising 40 minutes day by simply walking. After you feel that you are stronger build it up to an hour and more. Then you can kick up the intensity of the walk by utilizing a faster speed and going for a longer distance. Then add more days or exercise every day for at least 40 minutes. After 3 months of everyday training for 40 minutes you can start raising the stress level of your exercise again. Three months after raising your level of energy output, you may start increasing your time of working out. By then you will have increased your foundation of muscular strength and endurance and you will have done it reaping the full benefits as you have become healthier and wiser and much stronger.

EXERCISE PROGRAMS THAT CAN BURN FAT!

Warning: Before starting any exercise or change in nutrition you must check with your licensed physician and get cleared!

1. Martial arts, is a great exercise that utilizes your mind and body. Not only do you burn a lot of calories but at the same time but you also learn self-discipline and self-defense.
2. Swimming is a wonderful sport that involves all the muscles of the body and develops even the smallest muscle fibers that are used for speed.
3. Running or Power walking.
4. Sex is a very good way of burning calories and being intimate with your partner. Especially when love is involved and protection is used as safe practices are applied.
5. Aerobics classes and spinning classes.
6. Weight training. Use a medium weight for higher repetitions. Rest less between each set. Higher repetitions and lest rest make the workout more strenuous and burns more fat.
7. All physical activities involving more than on muscle group. Always with caution.
8. Work around the house or at work in accelerated pace.
9. Walking more and driving less when going to destinations needed throughout the course of the day.
10. Utilize less time sitting around and more time standing and moving around. Go out and leave the coach. A calorie burned is a calorie earned as a calorie not eaten is a calorie earned.
11. Be in motion and utilize different levels of speed.
12. Go hiking
13. Play safe sports.
14. Just move. The secret to all things is motion. If you move you need calories to move. If you're watching TV, use a hand grip or two. Think caloric burning with every action as you benefit from the reaction.
15. Think and be positive as you evolve in your sport and life.

THE IMPORTANCE OF EXERCISE, BOTH MIND AND BODY!

Why is exercise so important? Exercise is important because it helps you in every aspect of your life and at every moment as well. The food we eat is the fuel and the repair kit of our body. When we exercise the body uses the food it receives and converts it to fuel. This fuel is then used for our daily lives and our survival. When you exercise the body uses the fuel it receives and stimulates new repairs in your muscles tissues making them stronger and new cells for your organs making them healthier. Even though there are more things involved in the mix than just exercise, the utilization of oxygen is the start to all health. We call this cardiovascular training. It is the body's ability to utilize oxygen under different physical stresses at an accelerated and constant pace. When we exercise, our bodies use the fuel we give it according to the demands of the day. That is why it's always wiser to eat accordingly to the days demand for physical activity as oppose to a day of relaxation and just watching TV. Fat usually does not accumulate over muscles that are in constant use except in the case of obesity where the full body is affected. In obesity many factors take place for this disease. Our genes are one of these factors as well as our sensitivity and lack of self-control.

This means that the disease of obesity is more than just eating extra calories and limiting the use of those calories through physical motion. It means genetics are involved and a psychological factor as well. We will be tackling the psychological factor later. When muscles in the body are not used thru ought our daily lives repeatedly, the fat cells expand as the body stores the extra calories and distributes the extra calories according to muscular usage. As the calories or fuel go into the fat cell for storage, the cell expands and as it expands it traps water in layers as well as gas. That is why when you started losing weight in the first weeks you lose the most. Why? Well first, with the less food your intestinal track empties. Then gas is released and water retention which was trapped between the fat cell and the gas is also released. The tight bond that kept the layers affixed has been loosen with the cutting of the calories and as the fat cell has suddenly stopped expanding. But now instead the fat cell is releasing stored energy as it is now shrinking allowing the water and gas to escape. It happens at a faster pace when we exercise. Exercise stimulates the mind and the body together thru the utilization and deliverance of fresh oxygen. The fresh blast of oxygen helps the body utilize more of the oxygen, as the respiratory system delivers' it throughout every cell in the body and mind. Exercise helps you relieve stress and anxiety and forces more blood to move into working tissue, muscle and organs including the brain.

This provides the body with fresh nutrients and oxygen as vitamins are delivered throughout. When everything is working together your energy levels will be much higher. Exercise is such a key ingredient to overall health. When we exercise, we use up the waste in our blood as cholesterol starts dropping so blood flow can be increased. The benefits of exercise and cardiovascular training are limitless. Then why are we not all exercising? Let's take a look at the psychological factor behind this.

The reason why most people do not exercise and over eat is because of programmed responses known as habits that have been formed over a period of time with repletion. These habits that deal with different occurrences threw out the course of the day. We call these occurrences stimuli. These stimuli are what cause us to take an action to deal with the occurrence however these actions we try to make as painless as possible at the state of mind and body we are at the time. It all begins when we are children and as we are faced with problems we deal with them then in the mind state and physical state we are in as children. Other times we deal with the different stimuli by watching our parents or learning from TV. Repeating the same response to the same stimuli over a period of time and age, a habit is formed. Now we are older and are wiser and stronger being able to face similar stimuli differently. However we do not because we already have habits that deal with them created by us since childhood.

Now it's time to replace old habits with new ones that will motivate us and help us succeed beyond our wildest dreams. Everything we do in life is either to gain pleasure or avoid pain. We literally have repeatedly trained ourselves to focus on the wrong stimuli and to respond to them in a manner that is known to us and we are comfortable with. This has an effect on our day as well as our mood swings. Most of all we ourselves affect the way we perceive accept and think of ourselves as our ego and self-respect is constantly affected and challenged with the end results obtained from the wrong habits we have repeatedly executed. We either try to avoid the stress and anxiety of the day by eating, which provides us with a quick fix of pleasure. This fix usually comes in two different forms. This quick fix of pleasure comes by consuming food high in sugar or salt. This quick fix is usually in the form of chocolate, cake and other sweets as well as junk food or salty snacks. Why are these usually our choices? Very simple. When you are feeling down all these forms provide your mind and body with a rush or alertness as a quick pick me up. Just like caffeine and coffee does. All these stimulate the heart into working faster. When the heart works faster it forces more nutrients to go to the muscles and the need for more oxygen is increased. As the body rides the energy of the sugar or the spike of blood pressure from the sugar and or salt, we fall into a downward spiral of low energy and a drop in blood pressure that causes us sluggishness and a sense and need for rest or sleep.

When we exercise we force the body to respond with a natural high and peak releasing hormones and adrenaline and many other factors that cleanse the body, the mind and develop it as well as stimulating the production of new cells for our organs including the hair and skin. In other words from head to toe and all things internally benefit from exercise. When you exercise, you will force the body 99.9 % of the times into developing a higher level of fitness and well-being. By eating for a spike or high we force a temporary fix that stimulates laziness, fat and muscular cramping. This forces one into a state of shut down and a desire for sleep. The benefits of exercise are that it burns fat which is in the blood and the fat that is stored in the fat cells. The arteries and our heart are the pump and the delivery tubes, if you will, of the food we eat and the reserves that accumulate in our fat cells. If these delivery tubes our arteries are layered with blockage of fat and cholesterol, the pump that that is the heart needs to work faster and harder to force nutrients or fuel into the areas of the body that are requiring fuel. As the blood is forced thru the arteries it leaves behind traces or clumps of fat and cholesterol that are left behind and stuck to older deposits left inside the artery walls. As you can imagine the artery accumulates blockage and then unfortunately one day it closes completely. The heart tries to force the blood thru the arteries and the veins and works harder to keep up with your physical demands.

When the heart can't keep up with the body and minds demand for an accelerated deliverance of fuel because of blocked arteries, the blood flow stops, causing pressure and the blood then tries to flow back towards the heart instead of flowing away from it. This pressure causes a heart attack or an enfragma, a Greek word meaning fracture. Now the foods we eat are the causes of these clumps that are left behind in the arteries as well as heredity of higher triglycerides and cholesterol levels. This thick blood causes the heart to work harder or have a higher blood pressure than what is considered to be normal as the heart forces blood by pumping it faster to the areas that demand fuel while the muscles are demanding a faster and more powerful contraction. The bad circulation causes the body to tire easier and to be lazy and sluggish. The lazier the body gets the more it shuts down and becomes sluggish and the blood thickens and clumps as high fat and cholesterol flows thru the veins mixed with our blood throughout the years as the food we choose is digested and used. You might ask me? So how do we change our life and take control of our actions. We are so used to our habits and even though we want and desire change, we can't get ourselves to take new and appropriate actions. This is where your new formula and way of life takes up the slack and gives you a solution. Decisions plus actions equal change. To decide is to turn away from all other possibilities to take a specific new action which is a new choice to accomplish a new change and become a whole new you. This formula can be used in every aspect of your life to accomplish all new changes and start erasing old habits and replacing them with new ones.

This is a training formula that is simple and direct and it will help you reprogram old habits and replace them with new ones. Let's begin our journey now into a present and future that is all new and successful beyond your wildest dreams. Here is your formula to complete life changing success.

DECISIONS PLUS ACTIONS EQUAL CHANGE!!!!!

Decisions plus actions equal change. Wow! What a powerful formula yet so simple. In life all of our accomplishments were achieved the moment we made a decision and created the game plan for the actions necessary to make that decision a reality as we executed our game plan by taking physical actions. Whether that decision was based on avoiding or dealing with pain, or gaining and indulging in pleasure. Even if the decision was based on both pain and pleasure principals. To decide is to cut away from any and all other possibilities. Actions are the driving force that gives life to your decision and over a period of time provides you with a change in your life. Whether it's something added to your life or subtracted from your life, no decision can be enforced without physical action. Let's make a decision right now to change the quality of our lives by taking the actions necessary to lose weight and become thinner, fitter and healthier.

Let's start by deciding to train our mind and body utilizing the necessary techniques and taking the appropriate actions. To change old habits and create new and empowering ones is just a matter of replacing an old action with a new one. Repeat the action over a period of time and your result will be a new programed response to an old or similar occurrence and the erasing of an old habit. In the beginning when you are faced with a similar stimuli or occurrence you might need to pause for a moment and think of your new action and response as oppose to an old habit of response to the occurrence. This might be a little bothersome to you and you might feel a bit shocked or confused but remember that people usually avoid new actions and concepts and they run from them. Change requires to act based on a decision and execution of the action that is necessary, no matter how uncomfortable it may be. Break the habits that have held you back in life and have damaged your being and push forward into creating new habits that will empower you in your life. Always strive and push for success and you will succeed. The only things we can't accomplish or do in our lives are the things we do not want to accomplish or to do. We either take action or we don't. You are the master in control of your own life. Be a warrior and go into battle. Your brain is your greatest weapon and your actions are your sword. Believe me when I say, that all things in life are possible. Have faith and decide to believe this to be true for your life. I lost over 260 pounds and have kept it off for over 20 years. If I can accomplish this anyone can. Have faith and believe in yourself and your abilities. Keep your courage and be strong. Lead the way for yourself and then as a leader others will benefit from your accomplishments as well. Not by the things you say you're going to do but by the actions you take based on the things you say. It doesn't matter that I don't know you but I believe in you because I was once like you. I always tell people in my seminars that I was my worst student. Yet I kept striving and fighting for the new me that was hidden under a very big body and an emotional nightmare. Your decision to read this book alone shows me you are ready to take charge of your life and destiny. You are ready to live with no more limitations. That the new you is coming.

Have faith and believe in yourself. Everything in life requires faith and some form of belief. Faith is to believe that the actions you are taking based on your decision will result, in the accomplishment and gain of the end result. The end result was the thought that took place that drove you to decide to plan and to take action. Now you have gained and accomplished change. It all starts with a thought. All thoughts are brought to life with a decision, a game plan or road map if you will and with the physical execution called actions. Actions are that which brings all things to life and shapes your reality. Have faith and believe. Welcome change and challenges. Sometimes your faith and beliefs will be tested. Don't run from these tests. Fight and welcome them. Tell life to bring them on, at those moments you realize what you're made of and can become stronger and smarter as you defeat the challenge. Fight for your life and the way you want to live it. You are worth it and you get only one life. Seize the day and all the things the day brings so that you may learn and improve and succeed in all aspects of what we call life. No one will do it for you. It all depends on you.

For example: While exercising and eating wiser you may weigh yourself and have found to have not lost any weight. You become disappointed that you haven't lost weight and your faith is then challenged. Do not despair. There can be many factors that are causing the scale to be at the same weight. You might have water or soda bloat or you have added muscle. Remember that muscle weighs more than fat. Always strive and push forward by taking actions and sooner or later the actions will result in the accomplishment of your decision. Remember that if your actions are not getting you closer to making your decision a reality, don't stop and give up but instead just change your game plan and utilize different actions. No retreat no surrender. Never under any circumstances give up on living your life as you want to live it, in every aspect of it. Keep your faith and strive for your best results in all areas of your life.

Decide and act. Since we now know that we need to decide and to take appropriate action, why are we still procrastinating? Most people in life work themselves into a routine. They wake up one morning and notice that they have lived only a third of their life and now in their old age they feel that they haven't lived life to the fullest. It's never too late to decide and to take action. Routines are bad and most of us go thru life stuck in them or what others call a rut. We balance our lives daily into a 24 hour time frame. In those 24 hours we go to work and we eat. We come home and watch TV so that we may rest and then we go back to bed and start all over again. The moment we make a new decision and we start taking actions, our body goes into frenzy. We do not welcome and become very uncomfortable when new things are introduced to our daily routines. These routines have become our lives as we took the same actions over a lengthy period of time. These routines that are now habits hold strong roots in our being and subconsciously they have become your character. We follow the same routine over and over again and again as we become robots and a prisoner to our habits and routines. It's time to break free. How? Make new decisions and take new actions that will then give you change and a new happier, more successful and interesting, you. It is human nature that we live life as tolerable routine. Anything more than our routine is usually not welcomed by our body and accepted by our character. Take for example how you felt the moment you first realized you need to lose weight and started your diet? How painful was that in the past? The moment we say we need to lose weight or quit smoking or to change something, our body immediately goes into a lazy and uncomfortable mode. Who really wants to diet anyway? Look at the first three letters in the word diet. It states die. Subconsciously no human being wants to die and our brain is associating pain and discomfort immediately to the word diet.

Already we are in a subconscious bad frame of mind. We then build up the courage utilizing will power and we begin dieting and trying to do new things. We have temporary results and then we stop and one day go back to old habits. Why does this happen? This happens because we use will power. What is will power? Will power is the will to act without the basis of a decision. Will power is a force that will provide for you only temporary results. Will power does not give you the lasting result that a decision based action does. The changes that take place with will power become a lot more discomforting than a change that takes place thru a decision based action. These changes will not last as they are only temporary because your will and its power will sooner or later wear out. Actions based on a decision are permanent because you cut away from the power of your will and all other possibilities. That is what a decision is. There is no other choice when you decide but to be as you have decided to be because there is no other way suitable or acceptable to you. Will power on the other hand leaves a door open for escape. We all heard the phrase; I'm willing to try this or that or I might be willing to take up an exercise class. Decisions will sound like I'm taking and exercise class I'm doing this and I'm changing that no matter what. Do you see the difference? One is willing to the other is doing so. That is a big difference involving the human psyche. Will power says: I think I can do it and decisions say: I will do it. You must cut away from all other possibilities and make clear decisions as you execute appropriate action so that you may have the success you so desperately desire and deserve. You must decide and take actions daily to achieve success that will last a life time. This is the only way to reprogram yourself with new habits and create a look and a life style that is pleasing to you. You must cut away from all other possibilities and to do so you must make a decision and act on it daily. Even though there might be some discomfort at first remember that your old habits were not created in one day but over a period of time and repetition.

The same technique will now program new habits as your decision plus you actions bring forth a new life and new habits. Remember; if you have made any decision and are taking actions; notice the results of your actions. If you are getting closer to your goal then you know your actions are the right ones, if not and your results are not bringing your decision to life, and then just change your actions. You don't throw away your decision. Never give up or quit because that also tells you about and affects your character and how you perceive yourself as others watch your actions. In the bible God speaks of how a tree is known by the production of the fruit it bears. The tree is you and your decisions the fruit Jesus Christ our

Lord, speaks about in the bible is our actions. Decisions plus actions equal change. If all things in life and they are, as simple as making a decision, creating a game plan, taking actions with faith and belief and noticing if your actions are those that your decision requires for change, then why are we not all doing this in every area of our lives that we are unsatisfied with? Let's go to the next chapter in your work book so that we may get a better understanding of what I like to call the psychological factor.

DECISIONS PLUS ACTIONS EQUAL CHANGE. THE PSYCOLOGICAL FACTOR.

Let's start this section of the work book by making a list of all things that cause you to react or take negative actions when different stimuli occur during the course of your day and have affected your emotional states in your life. For example: anger, frustration, stress, depression, people and there negative remarks and everything else you find troubles you or affects you in a negative way. Next to this list write down how you have responded to these occurrences and the negative impact your old habits and or reactions have had in your daily life. Now sit back and notice how your old reactions and actions have led you down a path of unhappiness, weakness and low self-esteem. Now we must make a new list and change our actions to once that will inspire us, strengthen us and push us forward into becoming the people we know that we are and living the life we know we deserve. Once you have decided to change old actions to stimuli with new ones, the rest is just a matter of time and repetition. It is time and repetition that erases old habits and reactions with new habits and actions. Once you have decided on which new actions you will utilize in dealing with occurrences or life in general the rest is just a matter of repetition before you will have a new reprogrammed subconscious response.

This will have to be a daily conscious response until a new habit is formed thru repetition and time that will replace the old habit and response when the similar or same stimuli occurs now and in the future. Example: When I am angry I used to respond with unclear thoughts, physical strength and with a wicked tongue or by eating chocolate, drinking or eating junk food in large quantities while escaping into a TV world. Now the new me reacts to the same emotional state of anger by not going into a rage, by not using foul language by not over eating or drinking but instead with a pause. Then with an explanation to myself and the person who caused me to get angry, I explain what I'm feeling and why I'm feeling it and then with a work out, at a gym or a run to relieve myself of the anger. I help myself physically and mentally as my health benefits, instead of suffering with bad forms or unwise forms of abuse caused by your own hand. Do you see how the new actions benefit you when anger occurs as opposed to your old action or method of reacting to the same stimuli or angry emotion, which has driven you to a worst, physical and emotional state? Not forgetting that this old way of reacting with repetition over a period of time contributed to your character by creating a habit that was more damaging to you then benefitting you in every area of your life. Think before you act and react and just pause for a moment. Give yourself enough time to realize what your feeling and why and kick in a new positive reaction in dealing with the stimuli or in the above example, the anger.

This can be done with all emotional states and old habits as long as you decide to change and create new habits as you take actions. Use your mind and conscious thought. Think before you just act until your new actions become new subconscious responses and new habits erase old ones. Write down next to your old habits your new reactions to the same emotional states and decide to follow them from this day forth until they become a part of you and you need to think of them on a conscious level. This formula of deciding and acting to produce change works in every area and aspect of your life. Dealing with your emotions will become a daily focus in your life as your body and mind changes. The thought of food and exercise will be first on your mind because of the shock of changes that are occurring both physically and psychologically. In the beginning stages there will be times of frustration anger and mood swings. However stick to your plan and act on making your decision a reality. We all react differently as daily occurrences take place. We deal with these occurrences utilizing different emotional states of mind and body. These emotional states create a need to respond. It is natural to be tempted to respond to all stimuli with habits of the past. Even though it will be uncomfortable at times you must pause and take the time out to respond utilizing new actions that will push you to a successful change. It will become quite challenging at times however stick to your plan daily and you will be able to change your associations to the food and your old habits. Before you know it you would have replaced old habits with new ones, which will be making you healthier and more successful.

Our responses or reactions to different occurrences create a link mentally. We link emotions to the different occurrences and a reaction to rid ourselves from the mental and physical stress caused by the occurrence. Over a period of time, as similar stimuli are introduced into our daily lives our actions and or responses are usually the same. By taking the same actions we create a habit and a subconscious response to an occurrence as our mind recalls past actions taken that have had some form of dealing with, or have some level of success, with the occurrence. Also we link a way, to somehow deal with the emotional state using a physical means to relieve ourselves from the emotional and physical status that we undergo during our dealing with the different emotions we are under. Over a period of time, as the stimuli that affect us are usually the same, our actions and or responses are the same, which causes what is called a habit. These habits are a learned reaction to different occurrences daily. Now all habits are linked to 2 principals. To gain pleasure or to avoid pain and many times, to do both at the same time. Take for example how many times we have eaten something because we were either bored or stressed and even angry or disappointed. These different emotional states occur daily in once life since the time of birth. Since childhood even our parents have trained us by giving us candy or something to feel better when we were feeling down and when we did well in school for example our reward was food.

I remember my parents giving me some candy or a piece of chocolate so I can feel better when I was under stress. Instantly thoughts feelings or emotions were eased with the sensation of sugar or salt. Most of the time the foods are sugary or salty since the body craves them and loves them so much. So we start getting programed to want and expect and desire certain foods to make us feel better. Doing this repeatedly over a period of time, creates a subconscious desire and a response to different emotional states. Notice how we have linked food to give us pleasure and replaced feelings and emotions that are giving us pain, during the course of the day. This all begins since childhood. We are programmed that if we feel a certain way we eat chocolate or junk food and now we feel better. Now stop for a moment and let this sink in. Consider this. What would we desire if from the beginning as children, when we felt bad or suffered emotions or if we were happy our parents rewarded us with an apple or took us out for a run? Do you realize how important actions and reactions are and how everything is linked together? How many times did you eat when you weren't hungry but just under stress? How many times do you reach out for a specific food when you're feeling bad? These are old trained responses or habits when a specific emotional state of mind is occurring. A dealing principal to an uncomfortable feeling that replaces discomfort with a temporary fix of pleasure.

Now imagine if you will, what your life might be like if you had linked or trained different responses and had different habits pushing forward to better yourself in every area of your life. It's like a drug that one takes to temporarily ease a pain or suffering. Remember everything we do in life is to avoid pain and or to gain pleasure. Since we now have a better understanding about why certain desires arise without thought during different times or different emotional states. How do we change them? The answer is very simple. First we must be aware of that which is occurring to us at every moment of the day and how we are responding and dealing with the occurrence. We must make a note of our responses and if we are content with our habits of response. Once we know our selves then we can change our habits and learn to respond to stimuli with new actions repeatedly on a conscious level until the old habits are erased and the new reactions or actions become a new habit on a subconscious level. In other words, once we know ourselves, then we can change our habits and learn to respond differently. Imagine if we can respond to stimuli or occurrences with a programed subconscious reaction to the stimuli that pushes us forward to success. This creates a new you that succeed in such a higher level of success in all areas of your life.

Best of all imagine it happening automatically. No matter what is occurring in your life daily will be making you better, healthier, stronger and more successful. What a full and happy life that must be in all levels? Well, now it's possible as I train you and show you how to accomplish this level of overall success. Strive for leadership as you become the leader and the person you always dreamed and lead by your example as you become totally successful. Let's now begin! Grab your journal and a pen. Let's begin our road to complete success in all the areas of our lives starting first with our minds, body and health.

Decisions Plus Actions Equal Change! This is the secret formula and foundation to total success.

First decide right now that you are going to change your life and live it without limitations as you always dreamed of without settling for anything less than what you have decided. For three days right down in your journals everything you eat and drink. Write down the reason you are eating and the emotions you are feeling as you are eating. Even if you are feeling tired. After the three days you will get a clearer picture of your daily caloric intake, and the reasons you are eating what you're eating and how you are feeling as well. Once this is done start by making new decisions and what new actions you are to take at different emotional states. Also what type of foods would be a better choice? The three days are like a mini map or a blue print of your choices and habits. Now look over the three days. Notice if you ate because you were tired, bored, angry, stressed, depressed, upset etc.

In other words notice if your choices of food and the actual eating of food were for any other reason but feeling hungry. If so make a conscious decision not to eat unless you are hungry from now on. Look over the three days. Do you see any choices of food made were because of convenience or laziness on your part? For example: You were tired to cook and went by the drive thru at a fast food joint. Or your boss yelled at you and you ate a chocolate bar or bag of chips to feel better. You understand what I mean. We are not to eat unless we feel hungry and when we do eat we are not to get up from the table with a full stomach. Chew your food well and do not eat fast on the go or standing. It takes the stomach 20 minutes to signal the brain that an adequate amount of food has been received. Slow down and savor your meal as if it was your last. Eat only when you are hungry and never stuff yourself completely. Now look at the previous example about the drive thru. You could have made a choice of grilled chicken over a salad instead of a cheeseburger and fries. Taste is just a matter of getting used to. Don't use the example that one tastes better than the other. This is just an excuse. Use your conscious mind and take the necessary actions so that you may achieve maximum results. If you made a bad choice in food and not so healthy, don't scrap the day and say that I will start all over tomorrow and go on a sugar and salt binge. Instead just burn off the extra calories by cutting part of your next meal or exercising a little longer.

Don't fall into the habit of starting over and over again because that to, can become a bad habit and emotionally cause you anguish and a loss of your own self-respect. The time has come for a new life and a new you. No one will make the decisions and force you into action for you. This new foundation we are laying needs to be done with conscious thought and the desire on your part for change. It all starts with your decision to live a healthy, happier and more successful life. The actions of your choice will require repetition continuously so that new habits of success are programed and replace your old habits that have led you to the point you are now. If you don't start and carry out your actions now, if you don't decide and choose your new and more successful life now, then what are you waiting for? Every day that goes by is lost. Don't waste any more time. The new you are going to be amazing. I can't wait to meet you as well. Have faith and believe. Take action daily and never give up. Happiness is just around the corner. I know you can do it. Just do it already. Let's move on to the next part of our work book called breaking the pain barrier.

BREAKING THE PAIN BARRIER.

Once a person creates a habit and eases into a way of life he or she moves into a position of comfort and routine. The terms, this is who I am, or what can I do about it? Or I tried and I can't etc. are terms that people use to give themselves an excuse for giving up and not trying. One then reaches for a quick fix that usually comes from salt or sugar to ease the discomfort of lack of trying and say that they failed. All quick fixes' for one that is overweight will come first as food and then alcohol. People do this all the time to avoid pain or to gain a temporary fix of pleasure. To ease there discomfort and release themselves from feeling a specific or group of emotions. We do this so we can avoid pain and gain pleasure even for a moment, utilizing the 5 senses or as many of them as we can. Food is usually the first antidote chosen by people when they feel discomfort physically and emotionally. Why? Because food stimulates us utilizing our 5 senses. How? Let's start with smell. Which stimulates our mind and touch that stimulates our sense of reality by physical action. Then we have sight. Sight stimulates us by the appearance and color of the food as taste stimulates our glands. Then we have sound. We hear things cooking and the sound of a package of cookies opening.

All the senses work together as we are stimulated with the sound, smell, taste, touch and the appearance of food. That is why food is the antidote of antidotes. Besides the fact that we need it to survive, we use it to make us feel better as we abuse our caloric intake under different emotional states. The different emotional states are eased by the five senses that are being consumed with the food. By having the five senses occupied the body relieves itself from challenging emotional states by changing its focus. Once the focus is changed and the senses are occupied the body relaxes and the mind is at ease. Now imagine if we can instantly change our focus while under challenging emotional states and indulge our senses into a physical activity that helps you get healthier, stronger, smarter and even relaxes you? That is what a decision and the actions can do. You can actually train yourself and reprogram yourself to do anything. Instead most indulge in food to bury our discomforts, even for a short period of time. Usually after people are done with eating and binging they find themselves feeling uncomfortable and disappointed in themselves and their actions. We realize that more harm has come from the end result as we complete our binge or meal, than good because our actions have just driven us further away from our goal. We just used a replacement method that is contradictory to our decision to lose weight.

We replaced one emotional discomfort temporarily and have given ourselves another. Let's change from eating when we've had a bad day to exercising or reading a book. Use a replacement action that improves your overall being instead of one that cripples you. Be clear on what it is that you want and decide. Then take clear action utilizing conscious thought and choice as you bring our decision to life. Many times I have heard people tell me that they over eat, they make wrong choices of food and they do not even know why. Now you get a better understanding why and how to break old habits. Take actions that move you forward into succeeding in your new decisions and you now have progress and a new foundation of success and self-respect. Repeat the new actions over a period of time and a new habit is then formed. Replace an old action that drove you away from happiness and your desires as an end result, with a new one that brings you closer to the new you and your new decisions that become the driving force of your success. It's very simple to fall back into all habits because of repetition and training over a period of time. This is the reason why something new is inspiring in the beginning but we don't follow thru till the end because it becomes painful to act on a conscious and inspiring level all the time. Especially when you're tired and need to rest and are hungry and need some food. Who wants to put any effort under those circumstances?

If you don't put effort into yourself and your wellbeing, if you don't reprogram yourself for success and if you keep using the excuse that you will start tomorrow, your life will pass you by. You will never reach the level of success you desire and deserve. You will end up settling for the life and health you have in whatever little happiness you think you have. In time then you will break down further and realize that life has past you by and you have actually not lived it at all. The time to act is now. Take control of your life. Work for what you want and fight for the release and or reshaping of the new you. Decide and act. Decide to take control and be a leader and not a follower as you drive to success in every area of your life. If you do not then others will lead you and you will follow as emotions will lead you and you will grow weaker and unhealthier. Marketing techniques utilize repetition, emotions and your five senses to program you and train you on what to buy and what to eat, even what to believe. Stop being a victim to these expensive forms of programming and take charge of your own life. If you don't you will always be led and your habits and choices will be the ones that others have trained and programmed you to have. Be aware of everything that is going on around you. Jingles are a great programming techniques that teaches you to remember a product and to buy it. How many people know the sound of the ice-cream truck playing the same jingle over the years?

Need I say more? We hear the sound of the ice-cream truck and we instantly have the urge for ice-cream. This is just another form of programming using the five senses.

Everything worth having in life and not worth having requires a conscious thought and a physical action over a period of time. A period where the same action is repeated over and over again as the same emotion or stimuli is presented to you on a daily basis. How does one respond to a sudden occurrence or a repeated one? The first thing you do is pause. Ask yourself this simple question. The action I am about to take will it drive me further from my goal based on my decision or will it get me closer to my achieving it? At that moment you either give strength to your new life as you step closer to your new destiny and success or you will feel worse because you will fall deeper into your unhappy and unsatisfied life. You will feel incomplete and your self-respect and self-esteem will suffer. It's not that we are incomplete but we just can't help feeling as a victim of circumstance. Why? Because it doesn't matter who you are, we all carry the warrior instinct inside. The one that cries for justice power and respect. Including self-respect and accomplishment. Fight for the life you desire and demand. Take action. Never give up on your decision but simply fine tune your actions. Life is too short to be wasted on unhappiness and always wondering what could have been if only you had the nerve and courage to try. However, with obesity life becomes much shorter and depression a very powerful jailor.

Wake up pause for a moment and take conscious thought as you move forward to a successful and powerful new you. Every moment that goes by does not come back. There is no tomorrow, only the actions taken or not taken today. A calorie saved and not eaten is a calorie earned, used or burned off. You can make your change be less troublesome if you exercise more conscious thought, more actions and more self-control. After all I believe you are worth the very best this life and world can offer you. Get ready to receive it. Act now. All things are possible as the saying states. When there is a will there is a way. Don't forget I lost over 260 pounds and kept it off for over 20 years. Is it accidental? No way. It's a matter of decisions and appropriate action consciously on a continuous basis until the moment when it becomes a reaction on a subconscious level. I am not here to impress you or to brag however I am here to motivate you and tell you, that if I can do it everyone can. I just took it one step further and have become one of the best at what I do. Decisions plus actions equal a new you. We know have a better understanding on the powerful world of marketing and how repetition thru the years programs a person subconsciously and is responsible for the choices we make in life including food, clothes, jobs, vacations etc.

All these actions we take as we are subconsciously programed by movies and people are what develop our habits and character. Sometimes this is a good thing but most of the times it's a very bad thing. I heard many people say that they don't feel natural, that this is not who they are, why do I do this or why do I react this way. This isn't me. I have heard these statements over and over again. It is just merely knowing yourself and living free instead of being programmed and living a life with a subconscious reaction to all stimuli that has been imbedded in you utilizing repetition for a period of time. Fight and never give up. Stop being a victim and feeling sorry for yourself. Stop running away and hiding from this world. Others use drugs or alcohol to escape. Others have taken up smoking because of ads the cigarette companies have put out or because their favorite actors or even parents smoke. All these things are linked to first the 5 senses which is the door to the subconscious mind as it links emotional states to a physical action and reaction. In other words, you see your father smoking and because you love your dad and think he is cool you associate that feeling with the physical action of smoking without being aware of the reaction which can be heart disease or cancer. Another example is a relationship that ends badly and you are devastated. You might be crying!

That emotional state will link with other things happening around you that your 5 senses are tuned into. A good example could be a song playing in the back ground. Because you were in such a heighten state of emotion while that song is playing it links to your memory and your emotional state. Then lets same 10 years down the road you hear that same song playing. All of a sudden you get sad and your emotional state changes almost instantly and you don't even know why. You could have been happy one moment and then suddenly you hear the song and you just change completely and feel sad. Wow! What an anchor that is. Programmed responses that build your character and habits occur during heighten emotional states. It can be during or after pleasurable sex. Example: your partner will ask you for a favor during the moment of pleasure or immediately after your peak of pleasure. Nine times out of ten you will give into the request of your partner because of your emotional state which is at a pleasurable peak and then is linked to the feelings you have for your partner and for the favor they asked. Especially when love and feelings are involved. The foundation of programming is laid in one's subconscious mind during the time of heighten states of pain or pleasure. Good example during times of fear, pleasure, intimacy, satisfaction, hunger, happiness, sadness and mercy etc. While under extreme emotional states.

The brain and body are so focused and in such an alert mode that you can automatically link almost anything utilizing your 5 senses to that particular emotional state. Hormones and adrenalin are commanded to be released by the brain so that you may receive strength or back up for the bodies undergoing extreme emotional state. That is why, at that moment while undergoing a specific heighten emotion, you link subconsciously through your five senses to your brain a response or a way of dealing with your feelings or emotion as the body undergoes a hormone stability from your heighten emotional state. A good example of this is when you feel nervous and fearful at the same time. Then the stimuli or occurrence is linked utilizing the nervous system to every cell of your body. All stimuli are linked to every cell of the body thru the nervous system. That is why you can be fine and happy one moment and a single memory, word, song or image can trigger a sudden change in you. Then you are brought back to an old emotion and a feeling. It's like telling yourself over and over again that you can't do something or saying you hate a person over and over again. Then guess what? You won't be able to do it and you will hate a person because you have programmed yourself to do so. This how you can program and reprogram yourself when faced with different stimuli just by being conscious of what's going on and taking appropriate action as a response.

The rest is just repetition after a lengthy period of time at a heighten emotional state. Remember the door way to the subconscious mind is our 5 senses. Also remember that if you are not programming yourself by taking the actions necessary for your success in all areas of your life, then others are developing your character and your habits. It all begins from birth when the mind is wide open and we have no defenses. The mind at that age is like a sponge absorbing and linking thru the 5 senses and down the nervous system every occurrence with every emotion.

Now we have a better understanding about how habits, character and programming, form and shape a person to a life and destiny that might not be desirable. Heighten emotional states are very crucial to the linking of new triggers according to the stimuli presented. Now since we know how we are programmed during heighten emotional states and repetition than is it not true that we can do the same to ourselves with decisions and repeated actions of our choice as we stimulate ourselves into a higher emotional state of success? Yes it is true and we can replace old habits with new ones. Instead of reaching for ice cream when we had a miserable day we can now run for a mile. All it takes is the formula and sticking to your decisions by taking appropriate actions.

Instead of having a cigarette with our coffee we can have some fruit or cereal. Use a replacement method and just repeat the new action over and over again over a period of time. This way the old temptation and desire is wiped out as a new healthier habit is formed. It literally is that simple. Decide and act again and again until your new habit becomes an automatic response that is now part of your character and a new improved habit. To control one's self is to know one's self. Let's move on known to the following question. Why do we have such difficulty with new things and change? We know what we want to do or change. Why is it painful and uncomfortable to do so? Why such difficulty? It's called the powerful world of marketing and repetition. Linking thoughts emotions products to heighten emotional states. These are what we call anchors. We anchor emotions with a specific stimuli during heighten states of expression and feelings, utilizing repetition. We know have a better understanding on the powerful world of marketing and how repetition thru the years programs a person subconsciously and is responsible for the choices we make in life including food, clothes, jobs, vacations etc. We end up taking actions on a subconscious level that have been programed in us since childhood while we watched commercials and movies and listen to people we like and enjoy like singers, actors and athletes.

THE FIVE SENSES: TASTE, SOUND, TOUCH, SMELL AND SIGHT.

The 5 senses of the human body are responsible for all stimulation and all temptation. These senses are, taste, sound, touch, smell and sight. Let's get a better understanding on the powerful negative and positive affect our senses have in our daily life and how we can use them according to our plan of success. Let's start with taste first. Taste is the leading factor in choice making between one food and another or one drink or another. Basically everything that enters the body will be tasted and you will rate the taste of each thing that enters in and out of your mouth according to your own personal likes and dislikes. A lot of people automatically assume that healthier food choices, don't taste that good. That all depends on the preparation and once again changing old habits and desires with new ones that promote good health and weight loss while developing and toning muscles. We can substitute in the foods we love healthier ingredients that are better for us and lower in fat. Yes, the taste might change a little but focus on your end result and your goal. For example. Instead of baking muffins or a cake with whole milk, eggs and sugar, you can use applesauce, fat free milk and eggbeaters which are mostly egg whites.

There are so many healthier alternatives and replacement ingredients that can help you accomplish a well-balanced and healthier body that looks and feels great. Again, you need to decide and take appropriate actions. It's just a matter of training yourself and erases old habits by physically on conscious level take new actions so that you can, thru repetition create new habits on a subconscious level. These new actions based on your decision will provide for you a new life and a greater level of success, where you are in control. Simply put, if your actions until today provide you with a negative lifestyle or an unfulfilled one, then would it not make sense that if you did the opposite of what you have been doing you will get the opposite result. In other words, just change your actions. By taking opposite actions you get a whole other outcome. It's very simple. It's just a matter of making a decision and backing it with a plan and appropriate actions. Then the decision becomes a way of life as new habits are programmed utilizing repetition and time. Imagine if you do something and you don't like the end result just change the action and you will have success. It's all a matter of being aware of the actions you are taking and how they benefit us or hold us back in the different areas of our lives. This all intertwines with what we each consider success and happiness. What areas of your life do you feel need new decisions and new actions?

Sound and or hearing are another one of the five senses which promotes mood and causes the body to react with habits or actions. The things we hear can affect us either in a negative way or in a positive way. In the bible it states that faith comes by hearing. What we hear and what we allow into our minds is very important and must always be filtered. What we accept to come in will one day have a reaction to this action. A perfect example is a jingle. Have you ever heard a jingle so many times repeatedly over a length of time and even years? A good example is the jingle from the ice-cream truck. When we first heat it as kids or even adults on a hot summer day, we look to see where the noise is coming from. We then buy an ice-cream on that hot day that tastes good and we associate the feeling of enjoyment and relief to that jingle that we hear playing. A great example is the jingle from the ice cream truck or the church bell that rings at noon every day. This is all a matter of hearing the same thing repeatedly over a lengthy period of time. Then this jingle or stimuli becomes a subconscious automatic response according to whatever you associated or anchored to the jingle. If you were discussed you will hear the jingle and feel disgust. If you were happy then you will hear the jingle and feel happy but 9 out of 10 times if you hear the jingle of the ice-cream truck, you get in the mood for ice-cream and are ready to run to the truck as you did when you were a kid. It's all a matter of what emotion was anchored to the jingle. As soon as you tasted the ice cream and liked it, you just laid the foundation required for programming and the jingle was anchored as happy, yummy, musical and tasty ice-cream.

These feelings and emotions, anchor to the jingle as a positive emotional state. However, every time you went to the ice-cream truck you became a prisoner to your habit and subconscious response. The sense of sound.

What a way to program yourself subconsciously. It takes the human mind 6 repeated times, to hear the same thing, to start laying into memory, a foundation, of the associated stimuli. In other words, you hear the jingle 6 times repeatedly and it then starts settling into memory in your subconscious mind. Now the next part is what causes you to associate a mood or feeling to the jingle. What causes you to associate a feeling or mood to the jingle has to do with focus, your emotional state and the physical state you're in, when you first hear the jingle. Do you understand? Let's just say you're mad or angry. You hear a bad word used or foul language, or maybe you hear a specific song playing. Your mind using your nervous system instantly associates the way you are feeling at that high emotional state, everything coming in from your five senses. You will associate anger to the foul words and to that particular song. There are ways to immediately anchor a new action, when in a heighten emotional state and program a new reaction. The more senses being utilized at the peak of emotion, can instantly anchor a new response to familiar stimuli. Instantly one habit is replaced with a new response. We must always be aware of what is going on and what we are letting sink into our minds and bodies.

Think about how many things we hear over and over, again and again. Think about how these things have affected our emotional states thru out the course of the day. It's amazing how our characters and habits are formed by the help of others and our 5 senses while we are at a peak emotional state. If we are careful and know ourselves and our habits, we can become very successful, healthier and very powerful people in control of our own lives. We can truly be free. I once heard someone say that the mind is the most powerful weapon we possess and if were not using it to our advantage and programming ourselves to total success others will. The world of marketing is responsible for most of the programmed human minds across the whole planet. We are taught how to think, what buy, what to eat, what to wear and how we should act. The rest of our anchoring and programming comes from our parents, friends and our heroes. It all begins while we are still in our mother's womb. Successful marketing involves the usage of all of our 5 senses at the same time and are heighten emotional state. That is why TV commercials are so successful. Sound, to hear something over and over again. You have to remember that our minds is like a sponge and were programmed how to feel, how to act, what to buy, what to like, what to believe, what to hate and what to like. Imagine a world and a life where you are in total control and actually know yourself completely. Now the time has come where you are in such a higher understanding and you have been given a sword and shield to go and fight.

You can now understand how your mind has been absorbing information thru your five senses and has been linking physical reactions to your different emotional states. Over a period of time your emotions and actions are all based on habit. Habits that were created under false pretenses and were never your choices from the beginning. Now we can change all that since we now have an understanding and know how, to change. Imagine a world where you are in control of what we eat, what we do, how we feel, how we look and how successful we are.

Let's now move on to our third sense touch. Too touch and feel something is the ability to stimulate desirable trends and to be able to act on decisions. Touching something is the way reality or actions become more than just decisions, but become alive and even life in its self. By touching we feel by feeling we are stimulated by stimulating we act and react as we undergo different emotional states. By touching we feel by feeling we stimulate by stimulating we react. When we react we program ourselves under the 2 principals. Either pleasure or to avoid discomfort or pain. An example of pleasure when we touch is the softness of rose petals or our skin. The example of pain can be touching something very hot and burning our hand. During both occurrences whether pleasure or pain we link and anchor different emotions to the different stimuli. Thru out our lives we program ourselves to know that certain touches are pleasurable to us and other touches can be harmful and even fatal.

Touch is linked and goes hand in hand as all our tempting senses work together in full force. Continuous stimulation and temptation as our 5 senses work for us or against us. They are all based from decisions and actions. Act out your decisions with conscious thought until your repeated actions become a subconscious driving force of success in all areas of your life and not just overcoming obesity or losing weight. Imagine happiness and success on a level where the body reacts automatically as naturally as breathing, thinking, or as natural as your heart beating. These are some of the things controlled by your subconscious as opposed to your conscious thought. In life it is all a matter of deciding to do something and acting out your decisions with a clear game plan to achieve total success. Use your five senses for your total success. It is all a matter of deciding to do something and acting out your decision utilizing the power of your five senses as a driving force to a totally successful life. To each individual success and happiness comes in different forms. That is why it is important to make your own decisions and take appropriate action daily, for optimal and rapid success. After a period of time you will accomplish change. We all know what will truly make us happy. Go for it! We have a chance at happiness while we are alive and well. Let's not waste time. Let's make choices and decide to act now that you still can. If I could do it so can you. There is nothing you can't accomplish but the things you don't want to accomplish. I believe in you. Your destiny waits.

Our fourth sense we will be discussing is the sense of smell. How often are we stimulated by the sense of smell? Again the sense of smell falls under two physical and emotional reactions. Either as a tempter because we like it and enjoy its aroma, or as a rejecter because we dislike or despise its aroma. If you're thinking at this point, that we can reprogram ourselves to like what we dislike and dislike what we like, just by deciding and changing our actions and what we anchored to a specific emotion, I say to you congratulations because you got it. If food smells good we are attracted to it and smell causes us to feel hungry as well. However if something doesn't smell good to us, most likely we will not be tempted to even taste it. Smell is a factor that delivers a pleasing order or an unpleasant one threw out the mind and body triggering a response of pleasure or pain. The companies around the world have made lots of money producing perfumes and colognes. A great scent triggers a reaction of pleasure. Companies have made fortunes utilizing the senses starting with the sense of smell. Why? Because even with our eyes closed we can determine if we are going to like something or dislike it. Without even looking at it, tasting it, touching it or hearing it. We do not need to do anything but smell something and already we have laid out a foundation of like or dislike. For most people, that is enough. Sometimes we allow the other senses to stimulate us from a negative reaction to a positive one.

For Example. The food smells burned. So most likely we might not even try it. The chicken smells bad so let's not even attempt to eat it. The food smells, it's spoiled. I smell fire. However we might give in to the temptation of another sense. For example: The food smells burned. However the physical appeal is tempting because of the sauce that has coated it. Our five senses can be our best friends when they are working as tools to guide us in our life's decisions as we take action or they can be a destructive mechanism that will cripple us and keep us in a life of settling and unhappiness as we dwell in our limitations and programed habits. Smell is a very powerful tool because it causes the mind to release hormones that stimulate you and hypnotize you in a tempting way. You then react against your decision and take wrong actions or fall back into reacting with old unwanted habits. Be very careful to be in control and learn self-control. Don't be tempted to indulge in a subconscious desire to feel happiness or a temporary fix of pleasure. But instead take all actions to benefit your decisions and new life of total success. Look at relationships and how couples cheat on one another as they are temporarily stimulated by the five senses. Why does conscious thought lack a strong foundation?

Because we have repeatedly acted out against our decisions and have become slaves to our senses by giving into them and by accepting quick fix's during heighten emotional states. We either rush to receive pleasure or flee and give up so we won't feel any pain or discomfort. We have programmed ourselves unknowingly to be victims of circumstance and to give up and to give in to the stimuli presented to us thru our five senses. As others program us others program us and enslave us utilizing there expensive marketing techniques, we have become robots with characters and habits that enslave us to a life that is unfulfilling. We settle for that which we have been trained to accept and receive. We are victims of expensive marketing programming techniques and as robots we do things without knowing why. Automatically we tend to react without conscious thought, because we have been programmed thru repetitive actions to eat and buy and to react instantly according to the way we were trained by others and ourselves. The time has come to take control of our lives utilizing our senses according to our decisions and reacting with our new actions that will benefit us and provide us with total success. Then and only then can we be totally free and enjoy the fruit of our labor. Only then will you have true happiness and total success. Decisions plus actions equal change. Live this formula and you will be successful thru out your expectations. You will be successful at work, home and in life. You will lead by examples as all who know you watch and admire your accomplishments. Form new and inspiring habits and be a leader.

The world has enough followers. Have faith and believe in yourself and all things will be possible as your capable of all things. Remember your weapon which is your formula. Decisions plus actions equal change. Break the bondages you have surrounded your heart with and take charge of your destiny. Only then will you be truly free, happy, and totally alive.

Let's now move on to our last but not least, sense called sight. To see and to observe. We absorb in our minds in an accelerated pace everything that we are seeing. Now sight becomes even more tempting and powerful when it's used with the other senses. There is a saying that states the eyes are the mirror of the soul. Let's take a look inside, shall we? The eyes are the mirrors to the soul. What an interesting statement. Sight is one of the tempting senses because of the splendor of color and the visual affect from our color spectrum. The heart's desire is to see that which is appealing. It is in the beauty of all things that tempt us as long as it is appealing to us. Beauty is in the eyes of the beholder. Look how all things no matter how they smell or taste, if presented appropriately and with splendor, it will at least by tried or tasted. That is why first appearances and presentation is so important. The appearance and color raises interest and it draws the eyes for a better look. Then obviously the rest of the senses kick in as well but your curiosity has already been raised from the appearance. We as people are attracted to naturally to beauty.

Marketing agency's utilize this sense to draw attention to raise curiosity and to tempt all the senses. It's all in the appearance and the presentation. It all starts with the splendor and the spectrum of the eyes. The mind as I mentioned earlier, is a sponge. The eyes are also a sponge that absorb beauty, detail and at the same time brings out the hidden desires of your heart. Than many times those desires are acted out. We eat the chocolate or the slice of pizza even though we are not hungry. Once the heart is tempted and the mind receives a conscious thought of indulging or trying, the decision to lose weight or to achieve your goal should block out your desire to act. How? This is where the formula decisions plus actions equal change kicks in and will power is utilized temporarily to overcome temptation. Repeated it over and over for a period of time thru repetitive action and will power is then replaced with a new habit. Actions have results. From every action there is an equal or opposite reaction. Choose your actions wisely. Remember to not allow your senses to tempt you in any way and pull you away from your decisions and your actions. Your success is just around the corner and it should inspire you. Every time you overcome temptation you become stronger. Every time you give in to temptation you become a slave to it and lose a bit of yourself as you grow weak and weary. Before you know it you become weaker and you give up. Never give up on yourself and your dreams.

Every day or moment that goes by in once life is a fresh new opportunity and a fresh start. However every moment that goes by also never comes back. How are you utilizing your moments? Are they bringing you happiness, health and joy? Are they bringing success or financial freedom and are you growing as a person and an individual? Maybe your moments are bringing you stress, nervousness, anxiety, sadness, depression, anger and maybe even a lack or desire to live? Think about this carefully. Our actions are the driving force to our happiness and success. Your decisions are your focus and continuous perception on your life. Imagine your life where your actions are all based on your decisions. Imagine your life where your actions are all based on decisions you have made and are making. Imagine the happiness and success of a life like that. Decide to live a life of no limitations making every one of your passions and desires and every thought real. All this will be accomplished, by just making decisions and taking appropriate actions. Seize every moment because they slip away and never come back. In the lost moments, we lose out in our lives, expecting tomorrow to always be there for us. What if tomorrow never comes and your life has past you by and you have not even lived a portion of it to your fullest potential? By then it would have been too late. Stop living unhappily, stressed, angry, depressed and full of self-doubt. You doubt yourself already with the way you look, feel, and the things you do or accomplish.

With your choices of food, you can affect your life and jeopardize your health. That is why it is so crucial, that the foundation of the mind and body be solid. Upon that foundation you can program all new habits. Live and breathe. You are not alone out there. People are suffering even worse than you are. Please move ahead and just listen to the warrior inside of you and your coach. You can do this! It all begins right where you are. Your body is your vehicle that you will use for your life. Maintain, and turbo charge yourself. Don't crash your vehicle into a wall or a cliff. Decide and act! Enjoy your trip.

EMOTIONS: A DRIVING FORCE OR A DESTRUCTIVE ONE. CHOOSE WISELY!

Emotions play a very big role as every action is executed and we receive a reaction as the end result. Why does your emotional state drive you down a path that can be destructive or a path leading to success? The answer is the power of human emotion. An emotion is the root of every physical action and reaction. It is the driving force of all reactions that we take according to how we feel at the time that different stimuli occur. For example: You buy something you really wanted and love. As your holding it you drop it and it breaks or you lose it. Suddenly anger over whelms you and then sadness as the end result. Many people might feel more than two emotions going off inside them at the same time. Feeling these emotions your body wants to respond with a physical release. Your bodies discomfort might have been dealt with by eating, hitting or even yelling. In some cases you spiral down into a depressed state which is also a physical response. Discomfort can be characterized as anything that changes your mood from comfortable to uncomfortable throughout your day. To ease your discomfort you usually will respond with a physical action. At this point I'm sure we agree that an eating or hitting or yelling physical response is no longer required.

The actions you take during heighten emotional responses and discomforts are the most important. If when I'm feeling angry or upset, I reach for the chocolate cake, I would be responsible for driving myself into an unhealthy reaction to a discomfort or highly challenging emotional state. By doing so I'm training and programming my body to require and reach for a chocolate cake or other food when things occur in my life that makes me emotional or uncomfortable. I can easily go for a run or go shopping to produce the same affect the chocolate cake would have. The difference is with the chocolate cake I just consumed a whole lot of fat and calories. Instead if I went to the gym, I would have added to my fitness level or I could go shopping and reward myself with a new smaller pair of pants. One path and habit leads you away from your goal and the other path directs you to a better and healthier you. We have to understand that everything we do in life is either to avoid or to get over something that is causing us pain and discomfort or to gain or receive some type of pleasure and or satisfaction. However if I would respond to the emotional state of anger by exercising or reading a book for example, I have just bettered myself mentally and physically. One path leads you away from your goal and the other path directs you to a better healthier you. Why should I respond to any emotion with food or unhealthy other products. Instead I train myself to react with actions that will benefit the present and the future.

Once you realized and understand this fact you then have established the foundation of all human action and reaction and a better understanding of how our minds work and how we are programmed to respond with physical action and or reaction to the stimuli at hand. It is wise to stop and pause before we react and even speak. That moment of pause is important because you can introduce a new response or action with dealing with the occurrence and the emotional state. It's at those moments of conscious change that we start erasing old habits and begin laying down the foundation for new habits. For example. Your feeling upset or you just ended a relationship. In the past you might have responded to this stimuli or pain by eating ice cream or chocolate, maybe you like cheeseburgers or salty snacks. Whatever it was whether it was food or fits of anger where you break things, lead you down a destructive path and you have repeated this reaction or action to these emotions since an early age in life. Over a period of time you repeated the action or reaction, programming yourself subconsciously to respond this way to similar or the same, emotional states as well. Change your actions and the way you respond to different stimuli and you will notice that your emotions will change as well. Live life with a passion. All the control is in your hands. It is your reactions to your emotions that build your character and shape your destiny. If you have developed a habit that is bad, then to break the habit you must first decide to do so and then use a replacement method of response. In other words you change your actions. You replace one action that is new with the action that you would have taken in the past.

This way one old habit starts being erased and a new one being born. One way or another, all things in life is linked. Now that we understand and have realized how are 5 senses are the doors to all emotional states, we now can be aware on how to let thru the doors the things we want and slam the doors close on the things we do not want. You might be asking yourself how it's all linked together and how human emotion can make me unhealthy or unsuccessful financially or just plain feel a gap or un-fulfilled in areas of my life? Let me explain.

First we have our five senses or five doorways if you will. Through these five senses we receive stimuli, or bits of information. The stimuli or bits of information are processed by the brain and the brain sends signals thru the nervous system as a response. Either for the body to fight or go into flight. This bodily response is an emotion or a feeling. Once the emotion is triggered according to the stimuli, the body receives thru the nervous system a call to respond and act. We respond or take action in the manner we have programmed ourselves or others have programmed us to, utilizing repetition over a period of time. Repetition over a period of time is what forms a habit. To change the habit we must substitute a new response to the same emotions over a period of time. There is a way to erase an old habit and immediately substitute a new one. This again occurs in a high level of alertness and extreme emotional state. The way we react is a mere training principal or a continuous reaction and a repeated one. It takes the human brain six repeated actions to the same emotion, to lay the foundation for a new response and a new habit. After that it's a matter of repetition and time.

It all however stars with clarity, in other words knowing what it is exactly that you want to change in your life. Then it's a matter of decision making and appropriate action. The rest is repetition and a little time. The more one responds to an emotion with a specific repeated response, the more you give life and strength the habit. Once the action becomes a habit, your response to the emotion will be instantaneous. We need to pause for a moment and change the action so we can erase old habits. Just a simple pause is required to give in to the emotion utilizing old habits and you may then substitute a new action and response. Doing it over and over again, will create a new habit. Once it becomes a habit it is then a subconscious response. You will respond automatically in the positive and the old negative habit will have been erased. How many times have we reacted without thinking? That is because we have repeatedly reacted a specific way while under a certain emotional state. We repeated until it became a habit and a subconscious response. I reacted without thinking about it. It just happened. How do we change an old habit or subconscious response with a new improved one? Very simple. We use our formula for total success. Decisions plus actions equal change. First we decide to write down all the habits and areas of our lives that we want to change immediately. Then we write down next to them our new decisions and actions that will produce permanent change. We need to be very clear on what we want and what habits need to be changed. We must chose new reactions and put them into action utilizing repetition over a period of time until the new habits are formed on a subconscious level. Pick new actions that will better you in all the areas of your life, so no matter what the emotional state you're in, you will be benefitting continuously.

Let's use the following example. In your journal write and make a list of all the areas of your life that must be changed.

Lose weight
Exercise
Work Smarter not longer
Time Management
Stop getting Emotional
Stop having fits of Anger
Stop Smoking
Stop Drinking
Earn more Money

The list can go on and on!

Now let's begin with the first thing on your list for example losing weight. First you must decide to do so. Enough is enough. Then you must take the appropriate actions. Let's take for example: I must lower my caloric intake and fat consumption to (let's say your goal weight is 140 pounds) 1400 Calories a day and I must exercise 4 times a week for at least 45 minutes a day. The rest is simple it's the actual physical action of execution. Remember never to give up and scrap a decision to better yourself. Sometimes all you need to do is change your actions or fine tune them.

Please understand that every time you say you will do something or accomplish something and you don't you lose a part of your strength and belief in yourself. You start taking that which was once positive and turning yourself into something weaker and negative and then you begin reminiscing of who you once were and comparing yourself to who you now are that is unsatisfactory according to your own person beliefs and perception. After all, we are worst critiques. Let's stop this immediately. We are supposed to get better with age as a fine wine does. Not worse. Now your next step is the plan. How will I lose weight and become healthier. What actions should I take? Very simple. We know that weight loss comes from burning up more calories than you use. To expedite the process you can add an exercise routine. Exercising is not only great for burning calories at an accelerated pace but for also cleansing the body and mind. Exercise provides fresh oxygen and nutrients to the body in full and your circulation improves. Now the first decision is always the decision to decide to act. The rest of the plan has to do with the decision to take action. Wake up to this truth and decide right now. Life is too short to live it partially, unsatisfied and unhappily. Act now that you can so that you may live a life of success at the level you desire. Tomorrow is not promised to anyone. Let's live life with a passion and gain the fullness and happiness we know we deserve, with no more limitations. Imagine a life that you control your destiny. All the actions you take every emotion you have, all linked to positive reactions. Reactions that lead you to happiness, success and a life with no limitations. It's all a matter of decisions, appropriate physical actions and repetition. Imagine a life filled with only good habits.

Everything that has occurred in the past, no matter how painful or hard it was, no matter how many times you said you can't do something, or you can't stop eating and loss weight, let go of and bury right now. Every day alive is a fresh and brand new opportunity to gain and achieve total success. I believe that a person that tries and continuously takes actions and changes them according to their decision, will eventually succeed sooner or later. It will be just a matter of time. Even if the actions you take are not the best choices or not provided you with the immediate results as you change your actions the experience and the things that you would have learned thru the process are priceless. If you try something and it doesn't work, you must not give up. Just change your actions until you get the desired results. Never give up on your decisions and goals. Just fine tune your actions and learn from your mistakes. Nothing is a failure in life and there are no mistakes as long as you don't repeat them anymore and you have learned from them. Through the years you have made decisions and have taken actions. With some you have succeeded with some and others you scrapped as failures. You definitely have learned from both. The failures became failures because you gave up on them. Just change your actions, never through away your decision or your goal and mark it as a failure. The only thing we can't do is everything we don't want to do. Never give up and have faith. Believe in the unlimited abilities you have. You can accomplish all things and no things. You decide! The power is in your hands. Think about your so called failures for a moment. Have you ever realized the things you gained from the experiences? Think about your gains in knowledge and experience. What about your gains in power and strength to push forward in life and take certain abuses? That every time life struck a blow you are still standing. Does that not take strength? Yes it does.

What about your accomplishments? Whether you can admit it or not, you have gained though out your life with every action you have taken, at least knowledge if not more. All experiences some good some bad, are all gains at least in knowledge. There are no failures in life as long as something was learned or gained. Use what you have learned from the past to motivate you and strengthen you as you provide yourself with at least the hope for a much better future with no limitations. Have faith believe and hope as long as you are decisive and you execute appropriate action. The rest will be taken care with a little time. You must be patient. So believe in yourself and your abilities. Never say words like I can't do it, I'm not strong enough, it's so hard, I can't succeed because I'm a victim of circumstance. These are just all excuses to justify laziness and a lack of action. Be careful of the words that come out of your mouth especially when the concerned yourself. We tend to believe 95% percent of the things we say especially about ourselves. If everything you say is negative, sooner or later you will become spoiled and negative. If the things you say are positive and your actions as well are positive, then you will be fresh and be positive. What we say we believe and what we say programs us to act and helps us turn into what we want to be or what we think we are. Everything plays a role in your life including the people around you. Think about how often the people around you upset you or angered you. Whatever the emotions did you not consume food to get over your depression anger etc.? Most people utilize food 92% percent of the time to feel better. Is it an accident that junk food has such a big market? No its not.

We mentioned earlier that everything we do in life is either to gain pleasure or to avoid pain and even a combination of both. Well, sugar and salt are the antidotes. That is why junk food, candy, chocolate, cakes sweets, potato chips, ice cream etc. are consumed by people in such great amounts. Do you understand how everything in life is linked? Emotional states, negative results, beliefs, actions, reactions, faith, belief, words we say and others, the things we do and the things others do that affect us all these things keep us on an emotional roller-coaster. To all the emotions we link reactions based on our actions taken over a period of time utilizing repetition. We have created specific habits as we have trained ourselves using repetition over the years. To change our habits we must again execute new actions repeatedly. In the past we taught ourselves to flee and escape from our problems by eating sweets or taking drugs, by drinking alcohol and even making believe they don't exist by denying or running away from them. It's human nature to fight or to face things or to take flight or run from things. These are the 2 principals that all human psychology is based on, pleasure or pain. For every action there is an equal or opposite reaction. We must know choose our actions wisely. I know that it is about time we change our lives and live them to their fullest potential. To accomplish this we must first be aware of what it is exactly in all clarity, we want. Once we have done so then we can strategically plan our actions so that execution of them will be providing us with the basis of our new decisions. Then we can pause and not just react and substitute our new actions in place of the old ones. We now have the understanding and the tools necessary to react to the stimuli offered to us in life, through our five senses, with new actions.

By doing so repeatedly old habits are then replaced with new habits. Look at the example of anger. In the past you might have thrown something, yelled, screamed or buried yourself in chocolate. Now instead when the situation occurs you go for a run or for a walk. You read a book or have a conversation. You utilize new actions that will benefit you and empower you in place of old actions that harmed you and held you back. Deal with the daily emotions with new responses. A response that is positive and will help you in all areas of your life including your self-esteem. A response that makes you stronger and teaches you to succeed instead of one that cripples you and drowns you in sorrow. If you are training and programming yourself with new decisions and actions then all your life you will be left with the habits you have been programmed with by others since the day of your birth. Know yourself and who you are. You are the only one that can make yourself healthy, happy and successful. No one else can do it for you. You are the only one who knows what will make you happy and how. Decisions plus actions equal change. Be clear in what it is that you want. There is nothing you can't accomplish. Please believe me. Prove it to yourself or better yet see if you can prove me wrong. I challenge you to take charge of your life and become totally successful. As human beings we possess the most powerful weapon in the world. Our minds! Program it the way you want and the body will respond accordingly, as you gain total success in every area of your life as you live without limitations. To live without limitations is to live a free and productive life. I once heard in a movie, if knowledge is power than a God am I. Obviously we know we are not Gods. But God did give us the power of knowledge and the ability to gain knowledge.

However what is knowledge without action or a decision without action? Absolutely powerless. Nothing but a thought that blows away in the wind. How many times do we give others advice on what action they should take to resolve the issue, yet we avoid taking the same actions to benefit yourself, when the same or similar issue arises. Like that old saying. Take my advice please because I am not using it and please don't let my advice go to waste as I have. Take an infant for instance as an example. Tell the infant on a daily basis that it's lazy, until the infant grows up. The infant will grow up subconsciously thinking that it's lazy. The infant becomes a teen and one day an adult that will constantly think it is lazy. Words are very powerful so are beliefs. Repetition is the secret ingredient involved, in programming new habits and replacing old ones. Even old habits were formed utilizing repeated action. What do you believe of yourself? Do you use terms like fat pig, or ugly duckling, lazy or worthless how about weak and stupid, innocent, good bad? All these terms and others have been programmed in our subconscious minds as we heard them used repeatedly to describe us and others around us. We start believing them and we tend to use these words to describe ourselves during times of suffering and weakness as we are sad and feeling sorry for ourselves. Depressions then sets in and know we need to feel better. We then chose either a sweet or salty product or combination of both. By doing so we linked food as an escape from pain making it our reality and our way of dealing with, all things concerning our different problems and emotions. Do this repeatedly over a period of time and now you respond to those feelings automatically by reaching for a chocolate bar in order to feel better.

Can you see a clear picture of what is going on and how all things are linked? However now instead of heading for the fridge you go for a walk or a run. Now you just took a negative emotion and fed it a positive response. This is how you reprogram yourself. Where it doesn't matter what's happening in your life your actions whether conscious or subconsciously is leading you to success. All things are possible and nothing is impossible as long as you believe and have faith. First in yourself and then in me as you have hired one of the leading experts in the field of nutrition and fitness. Decisions plus actions equal change. This is the formula you need to achieve total success. Create for yourself a clear path of action to make your decisions a reality. After that it's as simple as taking the same actions repeatedly. Do not waste any more time and remember that all things require a clear and a specific plan of execution. The longer you procrastinate you are just holding yourself back from your dreams and your happiness. The past is the past. Let it go and start today as if you were born again at this moment. What matters in life is not what we have done but only what we do now. The now determines the future the past is just the learning experience. What we do now can be the difference between being happy or being miserable. It is all in the hands of the individual. I am happy that you have decided to go for it and create for yourself a new present and a successful future. Let's now move on to the next part of our work book called secrets and tips for a new and improved you. Use these tips so they can empower your decisions and give strength to your new actions.

SECRETS AND TIPS FOR A NEW YOU!

1. Never eat when you're angry.
2. Never eat when you're stressed out, upset or in a rush.
3. Never go super market shopping or choose to eat food that is not in your daily plan, when you are very hungry. We are led by our stomachs hunger pains, and our old habits kick into gear. As our actions come forth from our subconscious minds, and not our conscious mind followed by our new reactions.
4. Never eat when you're tired. The body responds by asking for food to keep energy levels up, and most of the time you don't require it.
5. Take up hobbies and occupy yourself and your free time with new reactions to life. Things which will help you improve your life and guide you forward to overall success.
6. Listen, we only live once. Is it wise to just eat and sit on the couch being miserable and in most cases alone while watching a movie and dreaming about a different life? Or do you think that you are worth actually living your dreams and having your old bad habits disappear one at a time? To be the person and live the life you always dreamed of can be a reality. The future is in your hands because the actions of the present shape the future. I made the choice and buried the old me. If I can do it so can you. I was my worst, laziest and indecisive student that I had the pleasure to coach.
7. React wisely to all temptations that come up against your new decisions. React by taking new actions based on your new decisions. React by taking actions that will benefit you immediately and in the long run.
8. Never react without thinking and pausing first. Your five senses can be overpowering and the temptations as well.
9. Utilize time to benefit the most out of everything you do. If time is money than life is time. Don't let it slip you by.
10. Always be ready to grow and better yourself. Learn to be flexible yet strong and direct.
11. Deal with the issues at hand. If something is bothering you, talk about it. Avoid letting emotions build up inside.
12. Remember you are not alone. No matter you it might seem at times.

13. Always study and learn new things that interest you. The more knowledge you have the better your actions will be to better your life.
14. Try to limit self-doubt about anything and find courage within yourself to accomplish all things that life brings before you.
15. Avoid negative people and surround yourself with people who are striving and succeeding and bettering themselves.
16. Avoid binging and over eating. We want to better ourselves so there are no short cuts. Vomiting and forcing yourself to do so is out of the question. That path leads to destruction and illnesses like bulimia and anorexia.

HERE IS MY SECRET TO KEEPING THE WEIGHT OFF!

I lost a lot of weight so far in my life and have kept it off. Even though it might seem to be a difficult task at times, I found that it's not. I am not telling you this to impress you but to encourage you despite your experiences and what you may have heard others say in the past about their struggles and problems concerning permanent weight loss. I lost over 200 pounds 20 years ago. I have been asked over and over again how I was able to keep it off. I found that permanent weight loss is just a matter of self-control with a twist of discipline. Imagine building a house on your own from the ground up and just when you're ready to move in you watch the house crumble down again before your eyes slowly one piece at a time. That is so painful watching your hard work, all the labor and sweat disintegrate slowly right before your eyes. Psychologically that is devastating as well and causes your self-esteem to drop tremendously in your own eyes. You believe less in yourself and abilities and enter a vicious circle involving a lack of personal faith. That's in the past. Let it go. Let's agree now as we decide and act that this will never happen to us again. So how do we keep the weight off forever? Self-control and discipline on your part and a weight loss / maintenance method that we call zig zag or to increase and decrease calories daily.

To keep the body in constant shock you must never let the body get used to the same amount of calories daily. This is the secret to maintaining your weight loss and staying healthy while at the same time your metabolism stays in a state of accelerated rate and is burning up calories as opposed to a slow metabolic rate. Decisions plus actions equal change.

The zigzag method to weight management is the action; the decision is to eat in moderation anything you want as long as your internal health allows you to eat a normal diet of course, is the decision. You don't have to eat everything in one day or in one sitting, no matter how much we like it. You don't have to burn yourself out in the gym in one day either. Use self-control and moderation for all things in life. Too much of anything is no good. There is a saying that states that Rome wasn't built in one day however it was destroyed in one day. Moderation is the key principal for all things in life. To moderately manage one's self in all aspects. To live affectively and truly be happy, in your life, involves a balanced lifestyle consisting of work, play, family time, exercise, romance and relaxation etc. If you only focus on work and is the only thing you do, you will miss out on other things in life. The same holds true if you only focus on playing. A well balanced life involves a combination of all things in moderation, just like weight management and health involves a moderation of a well balanced meals and vitamins. Moderation is the secret to total success and happiness, after decisions plus actions laid your foundation. The result is the changes and the happiness of a life that is totally successful that you decided on having and executed the actions to achieve it. Live life with no limitations and set no boundaries, however do all things in moderation and abuse no things.

Living a life till a ripe old age has no significance if you live it with limitations and realize one day you only truly lived a tenth of it. Don't wake up one morning with the thoughts I could have, I should have, I would have etc. Don't allow these to be your thoughts at a ripe old age so don't let life pass you by. Live for the day and better yourself always. Seize every moment as a fresh new opportunity and savor the gift you have. Tomorrow is not promised to anyone. Every morning think about the day and the things in life you want to accomplish that will bring you true happiness. An overweight body is a weak and lazy one that may cause you to lose out in life in general for many reasons including psychological ones.

The principals involving the zigzag method for weight management or weight loss, involves a daily caloric intake that will keep the body's metabolism from hitting a low or from going into a survival mode (which occurs with dangerously very low caloric diets and starvation diets). It involves a different caloric intake on a daily basis depending on the day's activities. To maintain a specific weight, it is wise to give yourself some flexibility which involves a 5-10 pound range, where you can fluctuate in weight for the rest of your life. Never exceeding the maximum gain of 10 pounds. This zig zag method of weight loss and management is a shock principal that never allows the body to get into any habit concerning caloric intake. The brain knows and learns that food will always be available and the body and the brain is justified and knows that it won't have to utilize or kick into a survival mode. Survival mode is when the body lowers metabolic rate to keep you alive and lowers the function or slows down the body's energy expenditure.

The way the method works is as follows. You set your goal weight at 190 pounds. That means a caloric intake of 1900 calories a day for maintained. One day you consume 2000 calories and the other day 1700 the following you might consume 2100 calories and the one after that 1400 calories. All the calories consumed for all the days on a weekly basis will average out to 1900 calories a day multiplied by 7 days giving you 13, 300 calories for the week. You can play with the calories daily. You can eat more one day and eat less the next day. As long as the number of calories consumed averages out to your caloric allowance for the week. In this case 13,300 calories for the week and every week to maintain a weight of 190 pounds. The changes in your caloric intake will go thru drops and peaks on different days. These high caloric peaks and sudden drops is the shock principal that stops the body from storing many of the extra calories as fat. It keeps your body's metabolism in high gear by not allowing the brain or the body to fall into a routine or habit of storing calories and slowing down the burning process. This way your metabolism is in constant shock and high gear. Take the daily calories and break them up into more meals and by doing so you will burn more calories and even some stored fat. In other words, the same amount of food you eat daily will burn more fat over five smaller meals instead of three bigger ones. Why? Because the body uses a certain amount of calories to digest the meal and your metabolism is in continuous shock from the food it is constantly receiving as it is mostly in digestive mode burning up calories and providing energy. Your body finds no need to store food in the fat cells because more food is constantly being made available. Life itself and all the things we do threw out the 24 hours on a daily basis, require a burning of calories.

Your body finds no need to store up food in the fat reserves or fat cells because more food is on its way and you have trained the body to know this. Everything we do in a 24 hour day requires a certain amount of calories to be burned. Your body is constantly burning up calories to stay alive. Now according to the muscular demands for fuel you can burn more calories in the hour of time or less. Let's take for example sitting on the couch and watching TV. You will burn in an hour fewer calories than if you were sitting on the couch watching TV and squeezing a hand ball and chewing gum all these things happening at the same time. Take the opportunity and utilize as much time as you can, burning off extra calories at different times of the day. Instead of taking an elevator for example use the stairs. Use your muscles and your mind. Train the body to work more and faster as every twitch of a muscle fiber or contraction burns off more calories and fat. The body has been created to take pressure and to be used. However the body has not been created to be abused. For every contraction for every breath we take or blink of an eye lid for every death of a cell and regeneration of a new one, a specific amount of calories is required. Since this is a fact and life maintenance requires water and food. The rest is just a matter of the bodies demand for fuel according to the minds command for physical motion. It's like a captain who is the head of his vessel commanding the ship to move. The head figures out what to do and your vessel follows the brains decision by taking action. These actions require fuel (which is food) and you are on your voyage in life. Everything we do, for every thought or muscular contraction at every moment since the womb we all required food. Our body couldn't even been formed without food in our mother's womb.

The zigzag method works wonderfully because it does not allow for habits or patterns to be formed concerning the same caloric intake on a daily basis. Since the body has been trained to know that it will get more food thru physical action, it finds no need to store a lot of food in the fat reserves. No don't misunderstand what I am saying here. The body will still store extra calories as fat however with the zigzag method it will store less and burn more calories than the average food plan because the body knows there will be more food available in a very short time. The water we drink daily, adds to this as well as our consumption of fiber, by flushing out and intertwining with excess fat and cholesterol. Then it all is flushed out as waste. If the average person wants to maintain a weight of 170 pounds, then that person will be consuming approximately 1700 calories a day. The 1700 calories a day when multiplied by 7 days gives you the equivalence of 8400 calories a week. The zigzag method gives you the flexibility of eating different amounts of calories a day as long as the total caloric count for the week adds up to 8400 calories. In other words, let's say on day one you had to consume 1700 calories and day two 1200 calories, then day three 1600 calories day four 900 calories day five 1400 calories day six 1000 calories and day seven 600 calories. The amounts of calories eaten for the whole week, once added up still equal 8400 calories. If you wanted to lose weight you can add exercise and you will lose weight or fat faster as the inches melt away.

However, if you are weight training to gain muscle you may increase your calories on the days you work out by having a protein shake that will provide with 30 grams of digestible protein after your work out and 1 more shake before bed. The shake should be low calorie and low-fat. I'm not saying that we should count calories for the rest of our lives. However we should be aware of them since the weight can creep back. Always remember that you must honor all your hard work and maintain your mental and physical transformation. Human beings have a tendency of forgetting things after a period of time whether they were painful or pleasurable occurrences. Being obese at one time is not something we should forget. Just like we should never forget what it took to transform our bodies and our minds as all the extra weight was burned off. It may start sneaking back on you slowly if you forget and are not careful. Besides the fact that obesity is a disease and can really affect your over health, wellbeing and shorten your life, it is something that can be repeated even after you have lost the weight. The reason for this is your body's ability to gain weight and the fat cells can expand again even after they were shrunk down with your weight loss. A fat cell can expand and can shrink. However fat cells do not go away or disappear. They are a part of your genetic structure. Just like the elasticity of your skin is. When you lose weight some peoples skin goes back into place hugging the muscles and others does not and you and up with lose skin that can be surgically removed. A good example is woman after their pregnancies. Other woman's bodies look like they never even gave birth because the skin went back to its original state and with exercise it tightened up.

Yet other woman still have the extra skin that hangs after they give birth and even though they lose the weight and exercise it never goes back completely to its original form. The skin is our largest organ and it stretches. It is unwise and unhealthy for you to always gain weight and to lose weight. It is best if you maintain your weight after you lost all the unwanted poundage. This must be avoided because it puts a lot of stress on your heart and your organs not to mention the mind. Remember that even though the heart is your strongest muscle, gaining weight and losing weight often especially large amounts of weight can be damaging to your heart and organs. Also the psychological factor is damaging as well. Yoyo dieting must be avoided for optimal health and weight management. When a person involves himself or herself with starvation diets, these principals of shock occur throughout the whole body. Besides the fact that even if the scale shows you losing weight you are mostly just losing water and muscle in a much more accelerated pace than actually losing fat. The body likes to be lazy and will take any opportunity to slack off so it may avoid wear and tear and prevent any uncomfortable circumstances. Let's look at this for a moment. We just had dinner and we ate some chocolate cake for dessert. The body has food to break down and digest for fuel however because of the chocolate and the sugar now available from cake it stores the food and uses the sugar for energy because it is much easier to use the fuel from the sugar instead of rushing to break down food and use it as fuel. The sugar provides the body with a quick burst of energy and the body then can take its time digesting the rest of the meal.

Once the body uses the calories in the sugar the rest of the meal depending on your demand for fuel will be stored and flushed out as waste. Most of it however will be stored as fat. This is just another reason why drinking a lot of water and eating fiber can be so useful. It prevents the body from storing all the extra calories and all the extra fat from the meal. Sweets and sugar is already in simple form. In other words it is predigested and goes right into the blood stream immediately entering your mouth from underneath your tongue. Since simple sugar or glucose is available, then why should the body rush and go through the trouble to break down your protein carbs etc. into glucose. It can use the sugar and digest the rest slowly as demand for energy occurs until the next meal. That is why you hear people avoid sugar and white flour when trying to lose weight including salt. Not to mention that sugar and salt open your appetite to eat while bitter and tangy dissolve your appetite. After all the body does not want to work harder than it has to. Look at how we get when we are tired or lazy and just want to lay on the couch and do something. Avoid sugar as much as you can and drink plenty of water to keep energy levels stable, to flush your body from toxins and waste and to help new tissue regeneration. Water is an important part of your daily lives so are vitamins are for overall health, diet and exercise. Remember to avoid sugar and white flour as much as possible and if you must have some, then make it at least 3 hours after your meal and limit your intake of the sugar and flour to one serving. Too much of anything is no good. Live life in moderation and always strive for unlimited success in whatever you do.

VITAMINS, MINERALS AND HERBS. IT DOES A BODY VERY GOOD!

Why are vitamins, minerals and herbs so important to consume daily with our meals? What's so special about them? Vitamins, minerals and herbs are helpers for the human body. Think of them as body guards and protectors that may stimulate energy, tissue repairs and a strong immune system to fight off disease and infection. They help regenerate new cells and damaged tissue and help in preventing the common cold by providing the body with more of a defense as they may boost the immune system into a higher defense mode. They are add-ons to make up for poor diets and lack of proper nutritional consumption. Vitamins, minerals and herbs are not to be used for substitution of food. We are living in times where there is a greater demand for food because of the planets population. Food in itself is not all being grown organically anymore because the soil and the regeneration of minerals in the soil, could not keep up with the demand for food quantities. Also let's consider how many vitamins and minerals are lost from just cooking alone. Think about how many oranges you must eat to consume 10,000 mgs. Of vitamin C. For most people the acid alone in 2 oranges would give them enough heart burn, imagine a case full and let's not forget the calories that come along with all those oranges. Vitamins are about adding on and not and not substituting.

If a person is on a crash diet or extremely low caloric diet, vitamins, minerals and herbs can be very important to help the body maintain health and energy levels. Please do not fall into the trap of extremely low calorie diets and crash diets. Avoid them like the plague. Vitamins are about adding and not substituting to a well-balanced meal. If a person is on a crash diet or extremely low caloric diet, vitamins, minerals and herbs may help you keep you going through out your day; however they will not prevent muscle catatrophy. I am really against low calorie and crash diets. However, vitamins, minerals and herbs can have an important role concerning overall health, wellbeing, energy levels and can help the body in every aspect. You can buy a complete vitamin and mineral formula and take the recommended tablet daily. You can increase your vitamin C intake and get an added burst of protection against the common cold. Like all things in life you should not abuse things and we should take vitamins, minerals and herbs as recommended on the label. Add the vitamins, minerals, herbs and enough water to a well-balanced diet or weight management program and you will find yourself functioning better in all aspects including a stability of energy. Water is very important so please remember to drink plenty of it. Coffee soda or any other liquid beverage does not take away from the water requirements daily nor does it makes up for a glass of water. The suggested amount of water daily as mentioned earlier is 8-10 glasses a day. You need more water if you're exercising and sweating and if you are consuming products with high amounts of caffeine.

When vitamins, minerals and herbs are used to add on, as oppose to a meal replacement or substitution, may provide you with better overall health and energy. Not to forget help strengthen your immune system. Vitamins, minerals and herbs may also help the body fight off disease and may even help the body heal faster. Think of a fine tuned engine which you take care of and maintain. You give it the best gas and then you add to it turbo boosters. Now you have a much faster more powerful engine. Vitamins, minerals and herbs are the turbo boosters, as the best fuel is the food you eat and the engine of course is our body. When all things are working at the same time, our bodies are faster, stronger, more powerful and energetic. Again remember that more is not necessarily better. Some vitamins are water soluble and any extra dosage or high doses that are consumed are flushed out without any damage being done to the body. Like vitamin C for example. Then there are vitamins like iron and zinc that if taken in high doses may harm you more than do you good. Please consult with your doctors before starting any new diet or exercise program. I also recommend a complete blood test and a stress test so that you and your doctor may have a clear picture of what is going on inside the body. These tests will help you identify your immediate health and you will get a clear picture of your internal health. Whatever you do in life, do it as well as possible striving for the best and do it properly. With every decision there is an action or actions that are necessary to achieve total success. This is your plan and road map. Decisions plus actions equal change. The plan itself and the execution of the plan, and the accomplishments thereof, are all actions that give life and meaning to your decisions. If a decision is the foundation than actions are the building blocks.

However we all still need the blue print, which is a clear plan of what the decisions will be and the actions necessary to accomplish your goals and plans. Even the plan is still an action as creating one to change your life is a decision. Always remember to follow thru and never give up on your decisions. Instead, always fine tune your actions in order to make your decisions while utilizing repetition a permanent way of life and success. Without a clear plan of actions you will take longer to accomplish your goals and bring your decisions to life. Let your first decision be to create a clear and direct plan of success.

Many times we hear people speak about losing weight for a specific event and we starve ourselves to fit into a dress or a suit. After the event we go back to our old habits and again the weight comes back because we haven't changed anything and have not created new habits. We have accomplished temporary results due to our will power and all of our work was in vein. The results were like a dream and the reality is that the weight comes back worse than before and you way weigh more than before. How do we make the results last when we take the weight off? Very simple. We decide and take realistic actions daily to accomplish new habits and a new way of life. We make all our new actions grow roots in our daily lives and over a period a period of time the repeated actions will become new habits that will guide you down a path of total success. Decisions plus actions equal change. What an easy formula and guideline to help everyone and anyone succeed in every aspect of their life. Have faith and believe in yourself and abilities. You may just surprise yourself and abilities. You may just surprise yourself and be amazed at what you can really do.

Obesity is a fast growing problem around the world. Especially with children. Technology has taken a lot of the physical activity out of everyone's lives, especially children. We need to stop this and return to old roots that required more physical action and play instead of sitting in front of a TV playing video games or on the computer. We can even drive less and walk more. We can use stairs instead of always taking the elevator. We can go and shop at a physical location instead of shopping online. In a world of convenience we suffer with obesity because we lack physical actions. Children can join sports teams and can help mom and dad around the home. The secret is physical activity. The more the activity requires energy the more the calories burned. Movement helps burn calories. The more strenuous the movement the more calories are burned. Movement that helps burn calories helps in all areas of the body. The more actions the body takes, the stronger it gets after time of recuperation. Sometimes we might feel discomfort and occasionally sore however the body will heal and you will get stronger. I remember reading once a slogan on a poster outside a marine recruitment center. It said that pain is nothing but weakness leaving the body. I remember thinking how true that statement is. It's fascinating to me how we really have no limitations as human beings and no crutches except for the ones we place on ourselves and death of course. Imagine a positive life full of success. It starts with a simple formula. Decisions plus actions equal change. It all starts with one decision. Decide to decide and to act.

I WANT TO LOSE WEIGHT HEALTHY AND FAST! JUST THE FACTS!

If you are like most people, than you want to lose weight as fast as you can. To feel good, look great and achieve maximum health and fitness levels is a life time commitment. However, if you were looking for quick answers and to wrap up everything up about losing weight and keeping it off, here it is.

To lose weight or to change anything else in your life you must first make a decision and cut away from all exceptions. Then you must create your plan in full clarity about what it is exactly you want to achieve and the actions necessary to achieve it. After that it's simply a matter of taking appropriate action daily, and continuously as repetition reprograms new habits utilizing your new decisions and continuous actions as the key to your new reality and life. How is losing weight and being healthy made easy? Very simple. First you decide to lose weight and then you decide to take action on a continuous basis for as long as it takes to achieve permanent change and results. Weight loss is very simple if you think about it in terms of simple arithmetic. If you eat less calories than you burn throughout the course of your day you will lose weight. The speed of your process is between you and your doctor as long as it's done with caution and overall focus putting health as a first priority. A healthy weight loss amount weekly would be anywhere from 1-5 pounds.

Avoid crash diets and metabolic shut down which usually occurs when the body goes into its starvation mode as a defense against very low and restricted caloric intake. Starvation mode itself is the bodies shut down of normal function, to protect and maintain life. It does this by limiting caloric burning and stores everything it possibly can daily, to maintain life.

This shuts down your energy levels and your activities are then limited because you feel tired and the body requires you to sleep. In starvation mode the body lowers your metabolism really low so that it can keep you alive as its main concern is brain and tissue function. In many cases it will even start breaking down your own muscle tissue and using it as food to maintain itself as it keeps the brain and organs working. You are to avoid falling into this trap. You might even think you're losing a lot of weight however you're probably losing more water and muscle instead of actual fat. Everything you do should be in moderation. Never use short cuts in anything you do in life. For every short cut there will always be a price to pay. People develop anorexia and bulimia because they eat and then go and rid their food by throwing it up using their fingers. Whatever you do in life try to does it right? Short cuts that involve the same old habits of over easting and lack of exercise result to temporary results and create health hazards like bulimia and anorexia. Bulimia and anorexia can be fatal. It is important to remember that everything in life worth having does not come easy. If it did than everyone would have it. However can everyone gain the same benefits in life? Yes they can. It all has to do with their decisions and their actions. Will all results be the same?

No of course not. We are all created differently with different DNA structures. Will we all gain results if our decisions and the actions were exactly the same? Yes you all would gain results, however the results would vary with each individual. Do you need to exercise? NO! It's a matter of simple arithmetic. Eat less than you burn and you will lose weight. Therefor if you are eating less calories than you actually need throughout the course of the day and you are accomplishing your goal then you need not exercise. If however you can find the time to exercise, I highly recommend it for many reasons. Exercise helps you lose more weight faster by burning up even more calories in a short period of time and an accelerated pace. Even after your workout you will be burning up more calories for hours than the average person who did not exercise. Exercise helps boost the metabolism into a higher gear. This simply means that exercise helps you utilize your food in a higher pace which is the explanation of metabolic rate. The metabolic rate of a person is their ability to utilize there caloric intake at a specific speed. Others have a faster metabolism, which means they have the ability to burn up the food they eat faster. Exercise helps boost our metabolism and provides the body with cleansing and over health. By cleansing I mean, the usage of excess fat and a cleansing of artery walls. This cleansing goes hand in hand with a low fat menu plan involving exercise, fiber, vitamins and water. When all these things work together your results internally and externally will be amazing. The following steps can help you maximize your results.

1. First decide to change your life.
2. Decide to act out your goal (take action) until you reach your goal daily and be constant in your pursuit.
3. Exercise if you can whenever you can. The benefits to your full body, especially your heart, lungs and brain are tremendous.
4. Write down in a journal 1 week's caloric intake so that you may get a clear picture of how many calories and what types of food you are eating daily. Also make a note during every meal or snack no matter how big or small the meal, what your emotional state at the time is. For example: I just ate ice-cream because I was upset and depressed or angry.
5. After the week is completed, look at all the things you ate and read your emotional states at the time you were eating them. Writing down I am hungry is not an emotional state but a physical one. Writing down I was angry is an emotional state of mind. Understand? Good let's move on.
6. Now notice all the times you were happy. Chances are that you were not eating unwisely at times of happiness and even maybe not eating at all.
7. Once you calculate all the calories daily and notice your pattern of when you're eating, what you're eating, what you're eating and why you're eating, you can start creating your plan for appropriate action. Know yourself and change what needs to be changed, physically, mentally and emotionally.
8. Once you decide on what it is that you plan to achieve create in full clarity a plan of execution and take the appropriate actions daily to achieve your ultimate success.
9. Weight loss is just as simple as eating less and burning more calories throughout the day and you will lose weight. It's a matter of simple arithmetic.
10. Have faith and decide on what it is exactly that you want and the actions necessary to get you there. No more thinking about it. You're

much better than that. You must act now. You can do it. Believe and have faith and act on a daily basis repeatedly.

Listen! If I can lose weight anyone can. It's all a matter of decisions plus actions and faith in yourself and your abilities. The end results will be amazing and your life will change for the better in all aspects. Just don't let all the attention you will be getting, swell up your head.

PUTTING IT ALL TOGETHER.

We now have a better understanding on how the body and mind works. We have learned how habits are formed and how we can easily change our old habits and replace them with new ones. All we need to do is to apply techniques that reprogram new habits under the supervision of repeated and direct actions. Use the formula and let it become a way of life with everything you do. Decisions plus actions equal change. We know how the body uses different food to help it heal and other foods for energy as well as the need for vitamins, minerals and herbs. We also know how to burn off calories and maintain weight loss. You can use the example menus in this workbook to help you and create a weight loss program made easy. The mind is a very powerful weapon and if you are not using it yourself the way you want under your control utilizing your decisions and executing your own clear actions, then expensive marketing techniques and others are using it to shape and refine you according to their own personal desires and needs. They do this by accessing your inner self and subconscious mind thru your five senses which are the doorways to subconscious and conscious thought. Let's put your new plan into effect. Your plan is your blue print for building your new self. Let's lay our foundation which is your decisions and finish building the new you. Remember that clarity on the specifics is the key to all decision making and taking appropriate actions that will drive you forward to all your successes.

First we begin with our formula Decisions plus Actions equal Change! Live this formula in every aspect and area of your new life. Consume it and make it yours. We can't accomplish permanent results nor take actions without decisions. To take actions thru will power and patience alone is a wasted effort that will provide us with temporary results and we will go back to our old habits eventually. To change all habits we must decide to do so and break away from any and all other possibilities. This goes the same for anything we want to accomplish in life. No retreat and no surrender is the focus and constant desire for accomplishing all new things. Live life to the fullest and don't let it pass you by. It will be a crying shame to wake up one morning old and grey and wonder depressed to yourself that if you would have, you could have and what if I did this or did that. Now once the clear decisions are made and written down our next step of the plan is to create a plan of actions. Again to do so our actions must be well thought, clear and precise done daily and repeatedly until they become a way of life. Now once we have our decisions the next step is the plan of action. The plan of actions itself is an action and has a foundation of strength. This is the basis of your decision. Never forget that if your actions no matter how well planned or how well executed they are, if they are not leading you closer to your goals, be flexible and just change them or fine tune them. Do not trash your decisions but instead just change your actions in order to accomplish your goals. You deserve the life you want to live the way you want to live it.

Step Two. We made our decision to lose weight. There is no turning back and we know have a clear focus and desire for the end result. Now we can create our plan to accomplish our weight loss goal effectively. Keep your work book handy and carry it with you. Let this work book guide you as if I am personally there coaching you. Thru this work book, I am there with you and coaching you thru all things every step of the way. Use this workbook as a guide to all decisions actions and successes. The plan calls for a low calorie menu plan and a realistic exercise program. Watch your fat intake and keep your calories based around your desired weight of achievement. If your desired weight is 160 pounds, than maintain yourself at an average of 1600 calories a day while utilizing the zigzag method I mentioned earlier in this work book fluctuating your calories daily but without going over the weekly amount which would be the total of all the days added up. That would be 1600 calories a day multiplied by 7 days in the week. It equals to a weekly goal and planned total of 11,200 calories for the week. My opinion however is that once you get an understanding of the amounts of calories you are used to consuming as you been gaining weight, cut back on them slowly and as your weight stars dropping you can then lower your caloric intake slowly instead of going for example, from 3000 calories a day to 1000. You can instead go down to 2600 for the first week and then drop down to 2400 for the next week etc. Use the zigzag method as described earlier and change your caloric intake daily but not to exceed weekly past the caloric safe zone. If you do so, make up for the difference in calories by exercising a bit more to burn them off. A calorie saved is a calorie earned. Memorize this phrase. A calorie not eaten is a calorie burned.

Don't abuse your body and over do anything. Instead use moderation and be patient as your life improves. Sometimes over doing things because you are impatient or in a rush can have the opposite results from those you are seeking. No pain no gain does not exist and in my opinion is a false statement and belief. Make things in life be fun and be creative. Only then can you learn and enjoy your progress and your growth as you become totally successful. You may use the sample menus that I have given you in your work book or just cut back on the amounts of food you are already used to eating. Try to lower your fat intake and cut back from the three whites. The three whites are sugar, salt and flour. In the beginning try to cut out completely sweets and sugar containing foods and drinks. At least for the first month. After that you may reward yourself with a low fat low calorie sweet twice a week and make up the difference in calories consumed with an extra work out, by cutting out something else from your food plan or by adding an extra 10 minutes a day for four days to your already existing work out.

Step three. What will your workout be? You must figure out which work outs feel comfortable and fun to you as an individual. The work outs must be safe and your body and internal health must be able to handle them without dangerous consequences. Once the body gets used to exercising you may then increase the intensity. Keep it simple and direct.

Make sure the workout is motivating and fun. Once you figure out what you would like to do in the form of exercise, and then put it into effect for three or four times a week as a start. I have found that as a coach my students are more inspired and excited when I use different workouts every time we meet. This way it is harder for them to fall into a routine and to get bored. Also using different workouts you get a better training of all the muscle groups in the body. The muscle groups can be broken down and include, small muscle fibers as well as the larger muscle fibers. Large muscle fibers are used to lift weights and carry you around. Small muscle fibers twitch or contract and are used for speed and endurance. The body has a tendency of adjusting to physical activity and caloric burning as it is only a matter of repetition that it requires to learn and adjust to new stimuli. That is why it's always wise to keep the body in constant shock. We do this by giving the body different food and caloric counts on a daily basis and changing the work outs on a daily basis. This shock principal keeps the body burning calories off at an accelerated pace as it learns new habits. At the same time it motivates and strengthens you to accomplish more physically as you continue enjoy the process of your transformation. Keep the body in shock and prevent it from falling victim to routine which leads to boredom. Use the zigzag method for burning calories or maintaining weight and change your workouts by alternating days and activities and stress levels. Do this and your body will be in constant alert and will not get bored or stuck in a routine.

Nor will it fall into a comfort zone and slack off. Instead it will lose fat and get healthier stronger and better as your overall health improves tremendously and in an accelerated pace. Please remember that you didn't put on all your weight in one day nor will you take it off in one day. Be smart and patient. Have faith and believe in yourself as the world watches and learns by your actions.

Step four. Begin programming yourself when the different stimuli occur daily by first pausing before any response and substituting your new actions instead of allowing an old habit respond as it did in the past. Remember think before you act and react because it is in those moment that new habits begin being programmed and old ones start being erased. Your actions shape your destiny while your decisions create it. Don't do anything in life dragging your feet. But instead face life and grab it by the throat. Be in charge of yourself and remember that every action has an equal or opposite reaction. This is a fact and is part of life. In the beginning of any new decision and action, once certain emotional states arise like anger, stress, fear, depression etc. human beings have a tendency of giving up and turning to some form of temporary relief. Then they want to give up and start getting depressed and feel sorry for themselves. Stop! Don't ever do that again.

Listen it's at the moments of heighten emotional states that if you take your new actions you become stronger and new habits are programmed much faster. Our reality or life is the result of our constant thought and focus. From this day forth make the decision to allow your reality to be a successful new you. Focus on your decisions and actions and you will have a new life as the old one slowly disappears. It is in those challenging moments that you need to keep yourself in control and think. Step forward at heighten emotional states and take your new actions and use them that are based on your new decisions. Be a leader because it's at those moments that leaders and egos and self-respect birth a new life for you. Step forward and seize your new destiny as you shape it and refine it using your own hand instead of letting others do it for you. Be the leader at least for yourself that you know you are. The only thing you can't do in life or accomplish is anything you don't want to do. No one is stopping you now so don't stop yourself and become your own victim and personal nightmare. Every day that goes by is a fresh new opportunity but every moment that goes by doesn't come back again either. Don't waste time anymore and bury your past know. The present and the future is the new you. It is in the moments of heighten emotional states that you can lay down the new foundation for new habits, and the old habits start disintegrating and losing their power over you. De root your old habits by not responding to emotions with your subconscious mind where your old habits have been anchored in repeatedly for many past years.

But instead pause for a moment and consciously choose your new action to replace your old one. Due it over and over again utilizing the same repeated action and response and new habits become a way of life as you reprogram yourself to achieve optimal success. Now that is a powerful new you. Troubles and emotions will always arise however, what shapes and refines you and your destiny as a person is the decisions and the actions you will now take. Human strength and abilities are shown during the hard moments in life. That is the difference between warriors and victims, between leaders and followers. If you keep on falling victim to your old programmed habits you will never reach your optimal success and be happy. The time to take action and show yourself and the world what you're made of is now. You demand change and know there are no more excuses. You know what you need to do and how to do it. Get up and do it. No one will do it for you, and life is passing you by. Besides, imagine the attention you're going to be getting from everyone that knows you and the world that lays eyes upon you. I know I'm excited to meet you and hear from you. Live life to the fullest and live life with a passion. Tomorrow is promised to no one so live today in total control of yourself by taking appropriate actions daily as you make for yourself a new reality and a new way of life. Take control of yourself by taking appropriate actions daily to make your decisions a reality as you lead yourself and others into a confident future with no boundaries no limitations and total success. I would love to hear from you and even work with you after your accomplishments.

In closing I want to congratulate you and even though I don't know you yet, I want to say that I'm proud of you. Your decision to seize life by the horns and live a life of total control of your being and reach optimal success in every area is exciting and inspiring. You have chosen to break free from your comfort zone and old habits that others have created for you since childhood. You have finally decided to break the chains that have bounded you for such a long time as your beautiful and sensitive heart has fallen victim to torment. Step forward into a new and exciting life that has no boundaries and no limitations because now you can make a decision and take action and accomplish your changes in all the areas of your life including financially. Have faith and believe in yourself and you will do it. If you're new actions are not getting you the results that you were hoping for, then don't throw away your decisions but simply just change some of the actions. You can do it. If you won't act now, then don't expect someone to do it for you. Take action with new actions as they are the roots that will help reprogram and erase old habits and install new habits. These new habits repeated over a period of time will create a subconscious response to different emotional states. A response that will benefit you in all areas of your life and you will be constantly succeeding. Depression, fear, anger and all other emotional states including old reactions will be ones of the past as they are now replaced with new reactions and actions. Your new actions will benefit you under strenuous emotional states. You will know that no matter what occurs in life you will respond according to your decisions and act accordingly to succeed fully. Your body and your mind will become stronger and your success will be evident.

Make a decisions that you will be not shaken or stirred nor will you be like a straw blowing in the wind waiting to break. Your decisions will have new strong and firm roots which will give life to your new you, as long as you take actions and thru repetition transform the quality of your life. Then after a period of time those roots planted will grow up in strength as you bring forth the fruits of your labor for the entire world to see. After all, a tree is known by its fruits. Is it not true that a human being is known by his or her actions? Absolutely a human being is known by his or her actions. Actions do speak louder than words. It is our decisions plus our actions that determine who we are and what were made of. Watch closely what you say about yourself and the things that come out of your mouth because it shows the world that you really are inside and what your heart is made of. Another reason you should watch what you say is because we have a tendency to believe the words that come out of our mouths. Especially if were criticizing ourselves. We tend to believe the things we say. If you talk badly about yourself and you believe the worst about yourself then you will live a life of depression and weakness. Sometimes in life it's just better not to say anything and just push forward with your actions as your decisions become real. A picture is worth a thousand words. Let your actions and accomplishments speak for themselves. Believe and have faith in yourself and your abilities. Make your decisions and create your clear course of action. The rest is just executing the plan. If your success or actions need to be speed up or fine-tuned, just change your actions. I will wait to hear from you and rejoice with you in all your successes. Good luck and talk to you soon. Live life to its fullest. Start now!

SAMPLE MENUS

Breakfast

1 bagel toasted
1 teaspoon of jelly
1 coffee black with fat free milk and sugar substitute
½ grapefruit
1 cup of water

Lunch

1 large salad
2 teaspoons of olive oil and 2 teaspoons of vinegar or lemon juice
1 glass of water

Dinner

1 Six ounce cooked hamburger made from 95 percent lean sirloin meat.
2 slices of whole wheat bread
½ a pickle
1 potato baked or baked fries one serving
½ grapefruit
1 eight ounce cup of diet soda

SAMPLE MENUS

Breakfast

½ a grapefruit
1 cup of coffee black or with a sugar substitute
1 cup of fat free milk
1 toasted English muffin with ½ a teaspoon of butter
1 glass of water

Lunch

1 large salad with 2 teaspoons of olive oil and a teaspoon of vinegar
1 diet beverage
4-6 egg whites
2 glasses of water

Dinner

1 small dinner role
1 serving of brown rice
1 serving of steamed vegetables
1 chicken breast broiled
½ a grapefruit

SAMPLE MENUS

Breakfast

1 bran muffin low fat or fat free
1 coffee preferably black
1 cup of fat free milk
½ a grape fruit
1 glass of water

Lunch

1 small fruit salad
1 serving of fat free yogurt
2 glasses of water
1 serving of pretzels
1 diet beverage

Dinner

6-8 ounces broiled or steamed fish of your choice
2 servings of mixed vegetables
½ a grapefruit
2 glasses of water
1 glass of wine

SAMPLE MENUS

Breakfast

½ a grapefruit
1 coffee black
1 cup of fat free milk
1 serving of cereal, your choice
1 glass of water

Lunch

1 English muffin toasted
2 slices of turkey breast
½ a tomato
1 slice of fat free cheese
2 glasses of water
1 apple

Dinner

6-8 ounces of broiled protein of your choice
1 small salad with 2 tablespoons of fat free dressing
2 glasses of water
1 apple

SAMPLE MENUS

Breakfast

½ a grapefruit
1 English muffin
1 teaspoon of jam or jelly
1 teaspoon of butter
1 coffee black
1 glass of water

Lunch

1 small fruit salad
2 glasses of water
1 cup of fat free yogurt or pudding

Dinner

1 beef patty 6 ounces cooked, with onion and garlic
2 slices of toasted light or fat free bread
1 slice of fat free cheese
½ a tomato and 3 leafs of lettuce
1 pickle
1 apple

SAMPLE MENUS

Breakfast

2 waffles
1 tablespoon of honey
1 coffee black
1 grapefruit
1 glass of water

Lunch

1 large salad with lettuce, tomato and cucumbers
2 tablespoons of fat free vinaigrette dressing
4 egg whites
2 glasses of water

Dinner

½ a chicken breast broiled
1 cup of white or brown rice steamed
2 servings of mixed vegetables steamed or boiled or baked
½ a grapefruit
2 glasses of water

SAMPLE MENUS

Breakfast

1 low fat or fat free muffin
1 coffee black or with 1 teaspoon of sugar
½ grapefruit
1 cup of water
4 ounces of fat free milk

Lunch

½ a can of tuna in spring water
1 small bagel plain
1 teaspoon of fat free mayonnaise or one serving fat free cheese
1 diet cola
1 apple
1 glass of water

Dinner

2 servings cooked pasta with one tablespoon of olive oil and garlic
1 grapefruit
1 large salad with 2 tablespoons of fat free dressing
2 glasses of water

SAMPLE MENUS

Breakfast

1 or 2 servings of oatmeal with cinnamon
1 glass of fat free milk
½ a grapefruit
1 coffee black or with sugar substitute
4 ounces fat free milk
1 glass of water

Lunch

1 small fruit salad
1 serving fat free yogurt
2 glasses of water

Dinner

4-6 ounces of cooked sirloin steak
½ a potato cooked
2 servings of cooked vegetables or raw vegetables plain
2 glasses of water with a twist of lemon

SAMPLE MENUS

Breakfast

½ a grapefruit
1 banana
1 orange
1 serving fat free yogurt
1 glass of water

Lunch

1 slice of pizza with your choice of 1 topping except extra cheese
1 diet drink
1 apple
2 cups of water
1 grapefruit

Dinner

6 egg whites
1 small lettuce and cucumber salad
1 tablespoon fat free dressing of your choice
2 glasses of water
1 apple

SAMPLE MENUS

Breakfast

2 servings of raisin bran
½ bananas
1 cup of coffee black or with sugar substitute
4-6 ounces fat free milk
1 glass of water

Lunch

1 small bagel
1 teaspoon of fat free cream cheese
1 teaspoon of jelly or honey
½ grapefruit
2 cups of water

Dinner

1 large salad
2 tablespoons of fat free dressing
1 serving of fat free croutons
4 egg whites
2 glasses of water with a twist of lemon

SAMPLE MENUS

Breakfast

2 rice cakes with one table spoon of fat free cream cheese
1 teaspoon of jelly or jam or honey
1 coffee black no sugar
½ grapefruit
1 glass of water

Lunch

4 egg white omelet with pieces of tomato, onions and I serving of mushrooms
1 serving of grated fat free cheese
2 slices of light bread or fat free bread
2 glasses of water

Dinner

½ chicken breast broiled
2 servings of mixed vegetables with no toppings
1 small salad with lettuce and cucumbers
1 tablespoon of olive oil and vinegar
1 glass of wine (not sweet wine)
1 glass of water

SAMPLE MENUS

Breakfast

1 low fat or fat free muffin
1 glass of fat free milk
1 coffee black no sugar
1 banana
1 glass of water

Lunch

½ bagel
1 cup fat free yogurt or light yogurt
1 apple
½ a grapefruit
2 glasses of water

Dinner

6-8 ounces of broiled fish
2 servings of raw or cooked broccoli
2 glasses of water
1 small salad with 1 tablespoon of fat free dressing

SAMPLE MENUS

Breakfast

½ a grapefruit
1 low fat or fat free yogurt with fruit
½ a bagel with a teaspoon of jam
1 coffee black no sugar
4 ounces of fat free milk
1 cup of water

Lunch

1 green apple
1 large salad with 2 tablespoons of fat free dressing
1 grilled chicken breast
2 glasses of water with a twist of lemon

Dinner

½ a grapefruit
2 servings of pasta or rice boiled with 1 tablespoon of olive oil
2 servings of cauliflower steamed
2 glasses of water
1 apple

SAMPLE MENUS

Breakfast

½ a grapefruit
1 coffee black
4 ounces of fat free milk
1 slice of whole wheat toast
½ teaspoon real butter
1 teaspoon of grape jelly or orange marmalade
1 glass of water

Lunch

1 sandwich low calorie and low fat with turkey (try subway)
1 diet soda
1 apple
1 glass of water with a twist of lemon

Dinner

1 broiled pork chop
2 servings mixed vegetables
2 glasses of water with a twist of lemon
½ a grapefruit

SAMPLE MENUS

Breakfast

4 egg whites omelet
1 ounce of fat free cheese
½ a tomato diced up
½ a serving diced mushrooms
¼ diced onion
1 coffee black or with sugar substitute
½ cup fat free milk

Lunch

1 apple
1 large salad with two teaspoon of olive oil or 2 teaspoons of fat free
    dressing
2 glasses of water

Dinner

1 or 2 slices of veggie pizza
1 glass of water with a twist of lemon
½ a grapefruit

SAMPLE MENUS

Breakfast

½ a grapefruit
2 servings of cheerios or bran cereal
1 cup of fat free milk
1 cup of water
1 coffee with 1 sugar or sugar substitute

Lunch

1 slice of veggie pizza
1 diet drink
1 glass of water
1 apple

Dinner

2 servings of pasta mixed with 1 serving of mixed vegetables
1 tablespoon of grated fat free cheese or low fat cheese
1 small salad with baby spinach and carrots
1 table spoon of fat free dressing
2 glasses of water

SAMPLE MENUS

Breakfast

2 pancakes medium sized
1 table spoon of maple syrup
1/2 a grapefruit
1 coffee black

Lunch

2 apples
1 banana
2 glasses of water
½ a grapefruit

Dinner

1 veggie burger
1 slice of fat free cheese
1 hamburger bun or dinner role
½ a baked potato
½ of a tomato and 4 leafs of lettuce.
2 glasses of water

SAMPLE MENUS

Breakfast

1 serving of oatmeal with a teaspoon of honey
1 coffee black
½ a grapefruit
1 glass of water
4 ounces of fat free milk

Lunch

2 slices of Low fat turkey breast with lettuce and ½ a tomato
2 slices of light bread
1 apple
2 glasses of water

Dinner

½ a Broiled chicken breast over a large salad with lettuce, tomatoes, onions
    and cucumber.
2 tablespoons of olive oil with 1 tablespoon of vinegar or lemon juice
2 glasses of water
½ a grapefruit

CLEANSING MENUS

Breakfast

1 serving of oat meal. With one teaspoon of honey
1 coffee black no sugar
1 grapefruit
2 glasses of water room temperature

Lunch

½ a chicken breast broiled
2 slices of whole wheat bread
2 leafs of lettuce and ½ a tomato
1 tablespoon of fat free dressing (your choice)
1 apple
2 glasses of room temperature water

Dinner

3 servings of boiled or steamed vegetables
½ a can of tuna in spring water
1 grapefruit
1 apple
2 glasses of room temperature water

CLEANSING MENUS

Breakfast

1 grape fruit
1 coffee black no sugar
1 plain rice cake
2 egg whites
2 glasses of room temperature water

Lunch

1 large salad with mixed greens
2 table spoons of olive oil
1 apple
2 glasses of room temperature water

Dinner

1 chicken breast broiled
1 cup of white or brown rice
1 grapefruit
2 glasses of room temperature water

CLEANSING MENUS

Breakfast

2 plain rice cakes
1 table spoon of fat free cream cheese
1 tablespoon of honey
1 grape fruit
2 glasses of water

Lunch

1 large salad with romaine lettuce and cucumbers
1 apple
½ a banana
2 glasses of water room temperature

Dinner

6 egg whites
3 servings of steamed vegetables plain
1 apple
2 glasses of room temperature water

THE 4 DAY WEIGHT LOSS SYSTEM

(Individual results will vary according to energy expenditure and metabolic rate. Average weight loss in 4 days will be from 2-12pounds. DO NOT REPEAT FOR ANOTHER FOUR DAYS UNTIL A THREE WEEK PERIOD HAS PASSED!)

DAY ONE

Breakfast

4 egg whites
1 coffee black no sugar
½ a grapefruit
2 glasses of water
½ a toasted English muffin plain

LUNCH

1 serving of fat free yogurt
1 apple
2 strawberries
½ a grapefruit
2 glasses of room temperature water

Dinner

4cups of steamed vegetables plain
6 egg whites
2 glasses of water room temperature with a twist of lemon
1 apple

THE 4 DAY WEIGHT LOSS SYSTEM

(INDIVIDUAL RESULTS WILL VARY. DO NOT REPEAT CYCLE TILL AFTER A 3-4 WEEK PERIOD HAS PASSED!)

DAY TWO

Breakfast

1 English muffin toasted
1 teaspoon of fat free cream cheese
1 teaspoon of honey
1 coffee black with no sugar
½ grapefruit
2 glasses of room temperature water

Lunch

2 apples
1 banana
4 strawberries
2 glasses of room temperature water

Dinner

6 egg whites with only pepper
2 servings of steamed broccoli plain
2 glasses of room temperature water

THE 4 DAY WEIGHT LOSS SYSTEM

(INDIVIDUAL RESULTS WILL VARY. DO NOT REPEAT CYCLE BEFORE 3 OR 4 WEEKS HAVE PASSED!)

DAY THREE

Breakfast

1 serving of raisin bran
4 ounces of fat free milk
½ a grapefruit
1 coffee with 1 teaspoon of sugar or sugar substitute

Lunch

2 glasses of room temperature water
1 small mixed salad with 1 tablespoon of olive oil and vinegar

Dinner

½ a grapefruit
2 servings of boiled pasta plain
2 glasses of room temperature water
4 egg whites

THE 4 DAY WEIGHT LOSS SYSTEM

(INDIVIDUAL RESULTS WILL VARY. DO NOT REPEAT CYCLE UNTIL 3-4 WEEKS HAVE PAST SINCE LAST!)

DAY FOUR

Breakfast

1 cereal bar
½ a cup of fat free milk
2 glasses of water
½ a grapefruit
1 coffee black no sugar

Lunch

1 slice of veggie pizza
½ a grapefruit
2 glasses of water

Dinner

6 egg whites
1 rice cake with I teaspoon of honey
½ a grapefruit and 1 apple
2 glasses of water

MY WORK BOOK NOTES AND JOURNAL

DAY_____MORNING

Upon Awakening I Create My Plan Of Action!

_____
_____
_____
_____
_____
_____

DAY_____NIGHT

The Actions I Actually Executed Today.

_____
_____
_____
_____
_____
_____

MY WORK BOOK NOTES AND JOURNAL

DAY_____MORNING

Upon Awakening I Create My Plan Of Action!

_____
_____
_____
_____
_____
_____

DAY_____NIGHT

The Actions I Actually Executed Today.

_____
_____
_____
_____
_____

MY WORK BOOK NOTES AND JOURNAL

DAY_____**MORNING**

Upon Awakening I Create My Plan Of Action!

_____
_____
_____
_____
_____
_____

DAY_____**NIGHT**

The Actions I Actually Executed Today.

_____
_____
_____
_____
_____
_____

MY WORK BOOK NOTES AND JOURNAL

DAY_____**MORNING**

Upon Awakening I Create My Plan Of Action!

_____
_____
_____
_____
_____
_____

DAY_____**NIGHT**

The Actions I Actually Executed Today.

_____
_____
_____
_____
_____
_____

MY WORK BOOK NOTES AND JOURNAL

DAY_____**MORNING**

Upon Awakening I Create My Plan Of Action!

_____
_____
_____
_____
_____
_____

DAY_____**NIGHT**

The Actions I Actually Executed Today.

_____
_____
_____
_____
_____
_____

MY WORK BOOK NOTES AND JOURNAL

DAY_____**MORNING**

Upon Awakening I Create My Plan Of Action!

_____

_____

_____

_____

_____

_____

DAY_____**NIGHT**

The Actions I Actually Executed Today.

_____

_____

_____

_____

_____

_____

MY WORK BOOK NOTES AND JOURNAL

DAY_____**MORNING**

Upon Awakening I Create My Plan Of Action!

_____
_____
_____
_____
_____
_____

DAY_____**NIGHT**

The Actions I Actually Executed Today.

_____
_____
_____
_____
_____
_____

TODAY I ATE THE FOLLOWING FOODS

DAY _____CALORIE TOTAL _____

A.M.

_____
_____
_____
_____
_____
_____

Total calories: _____

P.M.

_____
_____
_____
_____
_____
_____

Total Calories: _____

MY WORK BOOK NOTES AND JOURNAL

DAY_____**MORNING**

Upon Awakening I Create My Plan Of Action!

_____
_____
_____
_____
_____
_____

DAY_____**NIGHT**

The Actions I Actually Executed Today.

_____
_____
_____
_____
_____
_____

TODAY I ATE THE FOLLOWING FOODS

DAY _____**CALORIE TOTAL** _____

A.M.

_____
_____
_____
_____
_____
_____

Total calories: _____

P.M.

_____
_____
_____
_____
_____
_____

Total Calories: _____

TODAY I ATE THE FOLLOWING
FOODS

DAY _____ CALORIE TOTAL _____

A.M.

_____
_____
_____
_____
_____
_____

Total calories: _____

P.M.

_____
_____
_____
_____
_____
_____

Total Calories: _____

TODAY I ATE THE FOLLOWING FOODS

DAY _____ CALORIE TOTAL _____

A.M.

_____
_____
_____
_____
_____
_____

Total calories: _____

P.M.

_____
_____
_____
_____
_____
_____

Total Calories: _____

TODAY I ATE THE FOLLOWING
FOODS

DAY _____ **CALORIE TOTAL** _____

A.M.

_____
_____
_____
_____
_____
_____

Total calories: _____

P.M.

_____
_____
_____
_____
_____
_____

Total Calories: _____

TODAY I ATE THE FOLLOWING FOODS

DAY _____**CALORIE TOTAL** _____

A.M.

_____
_____
_____
_____
_____
_____

Total calories:_____

P.M.

_____
_____
_____
_____
_____
_____

Total Calories:_____

TODAY I ATE THE FOLLOWING FOODS

DAY _____CALORIE TOTAL _____

A.M.

_____
_____
_____
_____
_____
_____

Total calories:_____

P.M.

_____
_____
_____
_____
_____
_____

Total Calories:_____

TODAY I ATE THE FOLLOWING FOODS

DAY _____**CALORIE TOTAL** _____

A.M.

_____
_____
_____
_____
_____
_____

Total calories:_____

P.M.

_____
_____
_____
_____
_____
_____

Total Calories: _____

MY EMOTIONAL STATES TODAY AND WHAT TRIGGERED THEM!

DAY _____

TODAY I BECAME _____
_____
_____
_____
_____
_____
_____

I TOOK THE FOLLOWING NEW ACTIONS. _____
_____
_____
_____
_____
_____
_____
_____
_____
_____
_____

MY EMOTIONAL STATES TODAY AND WHAT TRIGGERED THEM!

DAY _____

TODAY I BECAME _____
_____
_____
_____
_____
_____
_____

I TOOK THE FOLLOWING NEW ACTIONS. _____
_____
_____
_____
_____
_____
_____
_____
_____
_____
_____

MY EMOTIONAL STATES TODAY AND WHAT TRIGGERED THEM!

DAY _____

TODAY I BECAME _____
_____
_____
_____
_____
_____
_____

I TOOK THE FOLLOWING NEW ACTIONS. _____
_____
_____
_____
_____
_____
_____
_____
_____
_____
_____

MY EMOTIONAL STATES TODAY AND WHAT TRIGGERED THEM!

DAY _____

TODAY I BECAME _____

_____

_____

_____

_____

_____

_____

I TOOK THE FOLLOWING NEW ACTIONS. _____

_____

_____

_____

_____

_____

_____

_____

_____

_____

MY EMOTIONAL STATES TODAY AND WHAT TRIGGERED THEM!

DAY _____

TODAY I BECAME _____
_____
_____
_____
_____
_____
_____

I TOOK THE FOLLOWING NEW ACTIONS. _____
_____
_____
_____
_____
_____
_____
_____
_____
_____
_____

MY EMOTIONAL STATES TODAY AND WHAT TRIGGERED THEM!

DAY _____

TODAY I BECAME _____
_____
_____
_____
_____
_____
_____

I TOOK THE FOLLOWING NEW ACTIONS. _____
_____
_____
_____
_____
_____
_____
_____
_____
_____
_____

MY EMOTIONAL STATES TODAY AND WHAT TRIGGERED THEM!

DAY _____

TODAY I BECAME _____
_____
_____
_____
_____
_____
_____

I TOOK THE FOLLOWING NEW ACTIONS. _____
_____
_____
_____
_____
_____
_____
_____
_____
_____
_____

IN MEMORY OF MY LOVING FATHER.

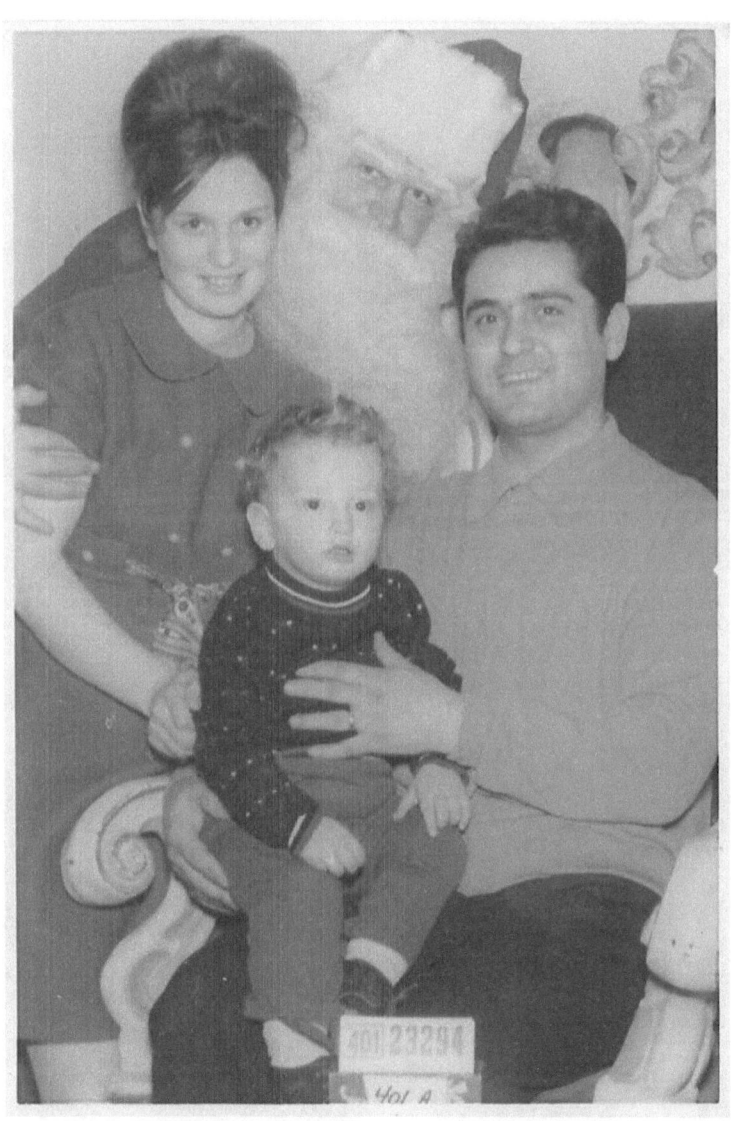

I MISSED YOU VERY MUCH.

www.ingramcontent.com/pod-product-compliance
Lightning Source LLC
Chambersburg PA
CBHW061307280526
45784CB00002B/921